NUMBER 728

THE ENGLISH
EXPERIENCE

ITS RECORD IN EARLY PRINTED BOOKS
PUBLISHED IN FACSIMILE

JOSEPH DU CHESNE

THE PRACTISE OF CHYMICALL AND HERMETICALL PHYSICKE

LONDON, 1605

WALTER J. JOHNSON, INC.
THEATRUM ORBIS TERRARUM, LTD.
AMSTERDAM 1975 NORWOOD, N.J.

The publishers acknowledge their gratitude to
the Syndics of Cambridge University Library
for their permission to reproduce the Library's
copies. Class-mark: Syn.7.60.45 and
Dd*.3.43^2(E) (pp: L_2v, L_3r, M_1v-M_1r, T_2r);
and to the Trustees of the British Library to
reproduce pp. A_3r, R_3r, R_4v, Y_4v, Cc_1r from the
Library's copy, Shelfmark: 1039.g.4(1) and
p. F_2r from the Library's copy, Shelfmark: 235.d.9.

S.T.C. No. 7276

Collation: A-Z^4, Aa-Bb^4, Cc^2

Published in 1975 by

Theatrum Orbis Terrarum, Ltd.
Keizersgracht 526, Amsterdam

&

Walter J. Johnson, Inc.
355 Chestnut Street
Norwood, New Jersey
07648

Printed in the Netherlands

ISBN: 90 221 0728 0

Library of Congress Catalog Card Number
74-28847

1941577

THE
PRACTISE OF

Chymicall, and Hermeti-
call Phyficke, for the preferuation
of health.

WRITTEN IN LATIN
By Iofephus Querfitanus, *Doctor of*
Phyficke.

And Tranflated into Englifh, by *Thomas*
*Timme,*Minifter.

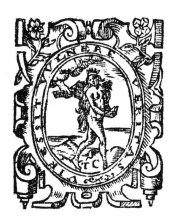

LONDON.
Printed by Thomas Creede,
1605.

TO THE RIGHT HONORABLE, SIR

Charles Blunt, Earle of *Deuonſhire,* L. *Mountioy,* Lieutenant general of *Ireland,* M. of the Ordinance, Gouernour and Captaine General of the Towne and Gariſon of *Portſmouth,* and the Ile of *Portſey,* Knight of the noble Order of the Garter, and one of his Maieſties moſt honourable priuie Councell.

 I may ſeeme (Right Honorable) an admirable and new *Paradox,* that *Halchymie* ſhould haue concurrence and antiquitie with *Theologie,* the one ſeeming meere *Humane,* and the other *Diuine.* And yet *Moſes,* that auncient Theologue, deſcribing & expreſſing the moſt wonderfull Architecture of this great world, tels vs that the *Spirit of God moued vpon the water*: which was an indigeſted Chaos or maſſe created before by God, with confuſed Earth in mixture yet, by his Halchymicall Extraction, Seperation, Sublimation, and Coniunction, ſo ordered and conioyned againe, as they are manifeſtly ſeene a part and ſundered: in Earth, Fyer included, (which is a third Element) and Ayre, (a fourth) in Water, howbeit inuiſibly. Of which foure Elements, two are fixed, as earth and fire: and two volatil, as water & ayre.

Geneſis.2.

That ſpirituall Motion of the firſt mouer, God, hath inſpired al the creatures of this vniuerſal world, with that ſpirit of Life (which may truely be called the ſpirit of the world) which naturally moueth, and ſecretly acteth in all creatures, giuing them exiſtence in three, to wit, ſalt, ſulphure, and Mercury, in one *Hupoſiaſis.* Mercurie congealing Sulphur, & ſulphur Mercurie, neither of them being without their Salt, the chiefeſt meane by whoſe helpe Nature bringeth forth al vegetals, Minerals, & Animals. So that of theſe 3. whatſo-

Eccle.3.

euer

euer is in Nature, hath his original, & is compacted of them, and so mingled with the 4. Elements, that they make one body. Therefore this Diuine *Halchymie*, through the operatió of the spirit (without the which the elemental & material Character, letter, and forme, profiteth not) was the beginning of *Time*, & of *Terrestrial existence*, by which all things liue, moue, and haue their being; consisting of body, soule, & spirit, whether they be vegetals, minerals, or animals : reseruing only this difference, that the soules of men & angels are reasonable & immortal, according to the Image of God himself, & the sensuals (as beasts and such like) not so.

Acts 17. 28.
1. Thess. 5 23
Heb. 4. 12.
Gen. 1. 16.
Wisd. 11. 17

Moreouer, as the omnipotét God, hath in the beginning, by his diuine wisedom, created the things of the heués & earth, in weight, múber, & measure, depéding vpó most wonderfull proportion & harmony, to serue the time which he hath appointed : so in the fulnesse & last period of time (which approacheth fast on) the 4. Elements (whereof al creatures consist) hauing in euery of thé 2. other Elements, the one putrifying and combustible, the other eternal & incombustible, as the heauen, shall by Gods *Halchymie* be metamorphosed and changed. For the combustible hauing in them a corrupt stinking feces, or drossie matter, which maketh thé subiect to corruption, shal in that great & generall refining day, be purged through fire : And then God wil make new Heauens and a new Earth, and bring all things to a christalline cleernes, & wil also make the 4. Elements perfect, simple, & fixed in themselues, that al things may be reduced to a *Quintessence of Eternitie.*

2. Pet. 3. 10.
13.
Apoc. 21. 5.

Thus (right Honourable) you see a *Paradox*, no *Paradox*, & a *Hieroglyphick* plainly disciphered. For *Halchymie* tradeth not alone with transmutation of metals (as ignorant vulgars thinke : which error hath made them distaste that noble Science) but shee hath also a chyrurgical hand in the anatomizing of euery mesen-
teriall

teriall veine of whole nature : Gods created hand-maid, to conceiue and bring forth his Creatures. For it is proper to God alone to create ſomething of no-thing : but it is natures taske to forme that which he hath created.

VVherefore if the foole which hath in his hart ſaid, *Pſal.* 14 1. *There is no God*, will put away the miſt of ignorance and infidelitie, and behold the power and wiſedome of God in his creatures, manifeſted more particular-ly, and inwardly by the Art of *Halchymie*, imitating na-ture in ſeperating from one ſubſtance, be it Vegetall, Mimeral, or Animal, theſe three, Salt, Sulphur, and Mercurie, ſhal by that miſtery, as in glaſſe, diſcerne the holy and moſt glorious Trinitie, in the Vnitie of one *Hupoſtaſis* Diuine . For the inuiſible things of God *Rom.* 1.20. (ſaith the Apoſtle) that is, his eternal power and God-head, are ſeene by the creation of the world, being *Col.* 2.8. conſidered in his workes. This Phyloſophy therefore (my good lord (is not of that kind which tendeth to vanity and deceit, but rather to profit and to edificati-on, inducing firſt the knowledge of God, & ſecondly the way to find out true medicine in his creatures.

Plato ſaith, that Phyloſophy is the imitating of God, ſo farforth as man is able : that we may knowe God more and more, vntill we behold him face to face, in the kingdome of heauen. So that the ſcope of Phylo-ſophy, is to ſeeke to glorifie God in his wonderfull workes: to teach a man how to liue wel, and to be cha-ritably affected in helping our neighbour. This Phi- *Gen.* 30.37. loſophy natural, both ſpeculatiue & actiue, is not only *Iob.* o.& 26. to be found in the volume of nature, but alſo in the ſa- *& 28 & .37.* cred Scripture: as in *Geneſis*, in the booke of *Iob*, in the 38.39. *Pſalmes*, in *Syrach*, and in other places.

In the knowledge of this Philoſophy, God made *Sa-lomon* to excel all the kings & Phyloſophers that were

in

in the world, whereby the Queene of *Sheba* was allured to take a long Iourney, to make an experiment of that wiſedome, whereof ſhe had heard ſo great fame, and found it by effect farre greater.

2. Cron 9.2
Mat 324.

Anaxagoras a noble gentleman, but more noble in wiſdome and vertue: *Crates, Antiſthenes*, with many others, contemned the pleaſures of the world, and gaue theſelues to the ſtudie of naturall Philoſophie. Philoſophers haue brought more profit to the world then did *Ceres*, who inuented the increaſe of corne & grain: then did *Bacchus*, that found out the vſe of wines: then did *Hercules*, which ridde the world of monſters. For theſe things belong to the maintenance of bodily life and pleaſure: but Philoſophy inſtructeth and nouriſh the ſoule it ſelfe.

This phyloſophy, together with the moſt rare, excellent & healthful Phyſicke linked to true grounds, and vpholden by daily experience, the very marow of true medicine, & the quinteſſence of marow it ſelfe, I moſt humbly preſent vnto your honours hands, as a Iewel of priſe, to procure and preſerue health: which *Ptolomeus* the ſonne of *Antiochus* valued at ſo high a rate, that he gaue to *Eraſiſtratus* a noble Phyſitian, on hundred talents for the curing of *Antiochus*.

My labour herein, be it but as the apple, which *Acontius* gaue to beautiful *Cydippe* to make knowne his amorous affection, yet being tendred with no leſſe good wil, in al humilitie I beſeech your honour to accept: hartily wiſhing that as you are a principal piller of this Common wealth, ſo it may be a meane to preſerue you in health with long life, to your countries good (as heretofore) and to Gods glorie.

Thus crauing pardon for my bold conceit, I euer reſolue to be,

At your Lordſhips Honourable pleaſure and
command, right humbly T. Timme.

THE FIRST
BOOKE OF THE PRACTISE
of Chymicall Physicke.

CHAP. I.

Ot only Hypocrates, but also all other famous Philosophers which haue succæded him, haue receiued their most principall grounds of Physicke & Phylosophy, from the Ægiptians. For the Aegiptians had a most singular knowledge of Astronomy and of the celestial courses, together with the vniuersal Science of the Mathematickes, and of such like Sciences. But the more general knowledge of all Sciences, is by Strabo ascribed, before al others, to that admirable Hermes Trimeg stus: as doth also Diodorus Siculus, who affirmeth, that the Ægiptians were the first inuentors of Sciences, taking their originall and infallible grounds from the same Hermes, or Mercury: whose diuine monuments are to be sæne at this day.

From this ancient Author Hermes, which liued in the first worldes, haue sprung vp all our Hermetical Philosophers and Physitions, whose traditions, haue bene receiued and imbraced, not only of all sorts of learned men in all countries, but also by the most noble and famous Princes and Kings, both Græcks, Arabians, and Latines.

Yet it must be confessed, that the most ancient learned Philosophers, neither haue nor could deliuer such a general knowledge, wherin there was not something wanting, and whereof themselues were not ignorant.

For (to vse the words of learned Guido) we are infants carried vpon the shoulders of those great and lofty Gyants, frō whose eminence we do behold, not onely those things which they saw, but many other misteries also, which they saw not. For no man is so sottish as to imagin that those first founders of Physicke had attained to the exact & perfect knowledge of Medicine, or of any other Science: which Hypocrates himselfe acknowledged in his Epistle to Democritus.

The same Hypocrates, howsoeuer otherwise singularly learned, and of all learned men for his monuments of Medicine, to be had in great reputation and reuerence; yet hath bewrayed his ignorance in mineralls, and metalline misteries: as appeareth in his booke of Simp. where he intreating of Quickesiluer, affirmeth that he neuer made tryall thereof, neither inwardly taken, nor outwardly applyed: bewraying his error in thinking that Hydrargyre, & Quick-siluer, were two seueral things : supposing that it was a medicine of Siluer dissolued into water, like vnto potable golde.

Hereby (I say) he hath bewrayed his ignorance in metalline substance, in that he knew not Hydrargyre, and Quick-siluer to be all one. Whereof neuer any man doubted, except he were so addicted to his teacher, that he wold say black is white, because his master saith so, which none of meane wit will do.

For as we thinke them worthy of blame, which with new found phantasies & toyes, do go about to burne & couer the errors of the reuerend fathers & ancients, as to many Empiricks and deceiuers, vnder the name and profession of Paracelsians: who also, do too stiffely and falsely ascribe to Paracelsus, as to the onely author, the knowledge of hidden things & causes, the finding out of mysteries, & the true preparation of al remedies and medicines : so in like manner they are to be reprehended which holde it sufficient, so as they talke of Galen without all reason, and affirme that he was ignorant of nothing, and that he came to the full knowledge of Medicine.

It is therefore well said of a learned & wel experienced lawyer, that it is a token of great rashnes, for wise men, either at the first to subscribe to error, or to subuert that which might

pleale,

pleafe, moderated with a temperate refolution. And yet learned men againſt all truth, do oftentimes barke againſt auncient wꝛiters, thinking it great honour and pꝛaiſe vnto them, if
they be able in any ſoꝛt to contend with their greatneſſe.

Thoſe Phyloſophers which haue wꝛitten of Chymiſtrie,
haue to maintaine their Science, Nature, Arte, and Experience : by auncient pꝛactiſe deriued from the Hebrues, Chal-
deis, Aegiptians, Perſians, Greekes, Latines, and Arabians.
This Science therefoꝛe is not grounded (as ſome ſuppoſe) vpon a vaine an imaginarie ſpeculation, but is found moſt certaine and infallible to the pꝛocuring of health, and length of
dayes to many, by the goodneſſe of Almighty God.

Neither doth this Science onely affoꝛd, common extractions of oyles and waters, by oꝛdinary Diſtillations, (as many
Emperits doe imagine) but alſo moſt pꝛecious Elipirs & Quin-
teſſences, much laboured, circulated, and wꝛought, by digeſti-
ous concoctions, and fermentations, by the meanes whereof
all impure and coꝛrupt matter is deſcked and ſeparated, the
euil quality coꝛrected & amended, & that which is bitter, is made
ſweet. Without the which operations, our bꝛead, beere, & wine,
the oꝛdinary and moſt pꝛincipall meanes of our nouriſhment,
become hurtfull & pernicious vnto vs. Foꝛ if we ſhould eat raw
wheate, oꝛ boyled onely in water : what & how many diſeaſes
would grow in vs ? Foꝛ this cauſe we ſeparate the pure from
the impure, that they may be pꝛofitable foꝛ vs, as the meale
from the bꝛan, the which meale oꝛ flower, we mixe with water,
we leauen and bake, whereof ariſeth a great magiſtery, namely bꝛead, fit foꝛ nouriſhment: and by his artifice, apt to paſſe and
turne into our fleſh: in the woꝛking whereof, if there be but a
little erroꝛ, it wil not be ſo pleaſing to the taſt, noꝛ ſo fitting to
nouriſhment, as is to be ſeene in bꝛead, either ill ſeaſoned, oꝛ
not wel baked: the which we reiect thꝛough theſe defaults.

The like pꝛactiſe & woꝛke is to be vſed in wines, if we deſire
to haue them fitie foꝛ our vſe. Foꝛ the pure muſt be ſeparated
from the impure, by boylings, digeſtions, and firmentati-
ons, ſeparating from the kernells and ſkinnes, the liquoꝛ of the
grapes, that it may be bꝛought into pure wine.   This

This done, and being put into veſſels, it woꝛketh newe ſeperations, fermentations, diſgeſtions, and purgations, ſeperating the dꝛegges and lees from the pure ſubſtance of the wine; the which ſo ſeperated, it becommeth fine and cleare, and is fit to be dꝛunke foꝛ nouriſhment: Whereas otherwiſe taken with the lees & not fined, it bꝛeedeth diſſenterie, fluxes, the ſtone, paine in the head, and pꝛocureth ſuch like diſeaſes.

Chymiſts therfoꝛe immitating nature in theſe kind of woꝛkings, and haue learned them in her ſchoole: finding by effect in natures woꝛke, that if common & oꝛdinary meates & dꝛinkes vnpꝛepared, vnſeaſoned, & rude, cannot be taken into our bodies without perill, then Phyſitians, and Apothecaries, ought to pꝛepare, ſeperate & purge thoſe ſimples which they ſhal vſe foꝛ medicine, by are ſeperating the croſſe impurity, that they may not be moꝛe hurtful to the weake and ſick, then pꝛofitable.

If Hypocrates oꝛ Galen himſelfe, were now againe aliue, they would exceedingly reioyce to ſee art ſo inlarged & augmented by ſo great and noble addition, and would patronize and vpholde with their owne hands, that which was hidden from the old fathers in foꝛmer ages: and reiecting many of thoſe things, which befoꝛe pleaſed them, yeelding to reaſon and experience, would gladly imbꝛace the new. Foꝛ it is euident by their wꝛitings, how vncertaine and doubtful they be in many things, by reaſon of the weakeneſſe of the foundation whereon they haue builded. Whoſe buildings notwithſtanding, vtterly to ouerthꝛow, no wiſe and modeſt Phyloſopher wil goe about, but will rather endeuour to vphold them, that poſterity may well and aſſuredly knowe that we were not barren, but endued with the ſame wit that they had, and that our mindes were ſeaſoned with that moꝛe noble ſalt. The which ſhall appeare, if not reiecting the wꝛitings of our elders, we ſhall inrich and adoꝛne them with newe inuentions.

Foꝛ artes come by tradition, and are deliuered as it were from hand to hand, and euery one adoꝛneth his arte with new inuentions, accoꝛding as he excelleth others in dexteritie of wit. And albeit, it may be ſaid, that it is an eaſie matter to adde to that which is inuented, yet both the Inuentors, and alſo the augmentors, are ſo be thankfully imbraced.

CHAP. II.

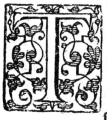 Here are thrée principall things mixed in euery Naturall bodie: to wit, Salte, Sulphur, and Mercurie. Theſe are the beginnings of all Naturall things. But he, from whom all things haue their beginning is G O D, vppon wheme all things do depende, hée himſelfe ſubſiſting by himſelfe, and taking the Originall of his Eſſence from no other, and is therfore the firſt and efficient cauſe of all things.

From his firſt beginning, procéedeth Nature, as the ſecond beginning, made by G O D himſelfe through the power of his worde. This Nature, next vnder God, aught to be religiouſly eſtéemed, thought of, enquired, and ſearched for. The knowledge hereof is very neceſſary, and wil be no leſſe profitable: the ſearche and raunſacking thereof wil be ſwéete and pleaſing. The profite which commeth hereby, appeareth in this, that the knowledge of all things which conſiſt thereof, and wherof they borrow their name and are called Naturall things, procéedeth herehence, whether they bée ſubiect to our ſences, or aboue our ſences. Hereupon great Philoſophers, both Chriſtians and Ethnicks, haue bene mooued to make the ſignification of the name of Nature, to fitte and ſerue almoſt all things. Inſomuch that Ariſtotle himſelfe, in that diuiſion which he maketh of Nature, diuiding the ſame into the firſt and ſecond Nature, and ſpeaking of the firſt, he calleth it Naturam naturantem. Naturing nature, by which he meaneth God. So in like manner Zeno, a Prince of Stoikes, openlie taught, that Nature was no other thing then God. Therefore the firſt Naturing nature is God; but the ſeconde which properly is ſaid to be Nature, is ſubdiuided into vniuer

B 3   ſal

Lact. lib. de
Ira Dei, cap.
10.
Plin. lib. 2.
cap. 7.
Sen. lib. 4,
de benef.
cap. 7.

(all and particular. The Uniuersall is that ordinarie power of God, diffused throughout the whole worlde, whereof it is layd, that Nature doth suffer this or that, or doth this or that, as Augustine teacheth in his booke De ciuitate Dei: and Lactantius: and among heathen wryters, Pliny and Seneca.

This vniuersall Nature, is also taken for the diuine vertue, which God hath put and implanted in all creatures: by the benefite whereof, certaine notes of the Diuinitie, are to be discerned in them. Hereupon some olde Fathers were woont to say, All things are full of Goddes, as did Heraclitus among others. Some others take this vniuersal nature, for a certaine influence and vertue, whereby the Starres do worke in these inferior things: or else for an acting vertue in an vniuersall cause, that is to say, in a bodie Celestiall.

Thomas lib. 9
super. 2. lib.
de cœlo.
Plato in
Timzo.

Furthermore, that is vniuersall Nature, wherof Plato speaketh when he saith: Nature is a certaine force and strength infused throughout all things, the moderator and nourisher of all things, and by it selfe the beginning of motion and of rest in them. The which Nature Hermes Trimegistus, almost in the same words saith, to be a certaine force risen from the first cause, diffused throughout all bodies by it selfe, the beginning of motion and rest in them.

This force the Pythagoreans called God. And therefore Virgil, a great follower of the Pythagorean discipline, wrote thus, saying: The spirit nourisheth inwardly, &c. And the Paltonicks called the same, the Soule of the worlde.

But yet the Platonicks haue not defined & shewed, in what maner, & by what means this Soule of the world, doth moderate and order all these inferior things, and doth stirre vp in the generation of things: neither can they yet determine.

But the more witty and learned sort of Philosophers, holde & affirme, that this world, which comprehendeth in the circumference and compasse therof the fower Elements, & the first beginnings of nature, is a certaine great bodie, whose partes are so knitte together among themselues, (euen as in one bodie of a liuing Creature, all the members doe agree) that there is is no one part of the parties, of that great body, which is not inlyned, quickened, and ſuſteined, by the benefite of that vniuerſall ſoule, which they haue called the ſoule of the worlde: affirming alſo, that if the bodyes of liuing creatures doe deriue life and beeing from the ſoule which is in them; the ſame is much more done and effected in the farre more noble and more excellent body of the whole world, by the meanes of the more potent and farre more excellent ſoule, with the which this body of the vniuerſall world is induced, and by which it ſubſiſteth. For if all the parts of the world haue life, (as manifeſtly appearing it hath) then muſt it needes follow, that wholely it liueth, for that the parts drawe and deriue their life from the whole, from the which they being ſeparated, cannot but periſh and die. And heereupon they inferre, that the Heauen compaſſing all things, is that Soule, which nouriſheth and ſuſteineth all things. Alſo, further they affirme, that all the formes, virtues, and faculties of things, by which all things are nouriſhed, ſuſteined, and haue their being, doe come from the worlds Soule.

And as the body and ſoule are gathered and ioyned together in one, through the benefite of the Spirits bond, for that it is partaker of both Natures: ſo the ſoule and body of the world are knit together by the meanes of the Æthereall Spirits going betweene, ioyning each part of the whole into one ſubſiſtence. And yet hereof we muſt not conclude as did Aphrodiſæus and Philoponas, which were Platoniſts, that the worlde is a moſt huge liuing creature, induced with ſenſe and vnderſtanding, wiſe and happie : the which is a moſt abſurde and falſe opinion. But the Platoniſts by the ſoule of the world, gaue vs rather to vnderſtand a certaine ſpirit, which chriſheth, quickeneth, conſerueth, and ſuſteineth all things, as it were a certaine ſpirit of that Elohym, or great Gen. 1. God, which moued vpon the waters : which Plato might remember, as one not ignorant of Moſes, and therupon frame his ſoule of the world. Whereupon alſo it muſt needes come to paſſe, that all theſe inferior things, otherwiſe tranſitorie and infirme, ſhould ſoone come to deſtruction, without they were

con

conferued and continued in their being by that diuine power, perpetually maintaining and fufpecting them : the which being diffenered , a great confufion & perturbation of the whole worlde arife therof. Which ruine and deftruction, God of his great goodnes would preuent, creating that vniuerfall Nature, which fhould defende all this great worke , and keepe it fafe and founde, by his vertue and moderation : and that by the yearely and continual rotation and reuolution of the right Heauen,and by the Influences and vertues of the Starres, Planets , and Celeftiall powers, all things might be well gouerned , and might conftantly remaine and abide in full faftnes of their eftate, vntill the predeftinated time of their diffolution.

To this Æthereall fpirit, or rather Diuine power, euery effectuall and Omnipotent , Plato in his Timæo giueth teftimonie, when hee fpeaketh thus : When the fempiternall GOD had created this Vniuerfal, hee put into it certaine feedes of reafon, & brought in the beginning Life,that he might beget with the world the procreating force. Wherin our explication which I brought before concerning the Soule of the worlde is confirmed. Which alfo agreeth with that which the Prophet Mofes hath written, and which King Dauid hath in his Pfalme, in thefe wordes : By the worde of the Lorde were the Heauens made , and all the vertue of them by the fpirit of his mouth. By which vertue of the quickning fpirit, that great Trimegiftus more conuerfant and exercifed in Mofes writings,then all other Philofophers, vttered thefe diuine wordes in his fecond booke,which is called *Afclepias* : All fpirit (faith he) in the world,is acted and gouerned by the fpirit. The fpirit telleth all things : the worlde nourifheth bodies, the fpirit giueth them foule. By the fpirit all things in the world are miniftred, & are made to growe and increafe. And after that he faith againe: All things haue neede of this fpirit For it carryeth all things, and it quickneth & nourifheth all things, according to the dignitie of eache thing in it felfe . Life and the fpirite is

brought

b?ought fo?th out of the holy fountaine. By which diuine wo?ds it appeareth plainely, that this eternall and quickening ſpirit is infuſed and put into all things : ſo that it is not obſerued to deduce and deriue the actions, fo?ces, and powers:alſo all naturall things,from the ſpirits,as from the cauſes.

CHAP. III.

Auing ſpoken ſufficiently of the firſt and ſecond beginning, that is to ſay of God & vniuerſal Nature : God the firſt cauſe vſing that generall Nature as his handmaid : it reſteth that ſomewhat be ſpoken of nature naturated,that is to ſay,of that which is particular. To make an apt and conuenient definition whereof, let vs knowe that it is no other thing , than euery naturall body conſiſting of fo?me and matter. Fo? of theſe two cauſes , and not onely of the cauſes, but alſo of the parts of the whole compound,all nature,that is to ſay,euery naturall body conſiſteth. Fo? the Peripateticks do thinke, that whatſoeuer is the beginning of generation, ought to be called nature by a certaine peculiar right. And Ariſtotle ſaith,that the ſame , from whence any thing is made at the firſt, and whereof it hath the firſt motion, mutation is the very beginning. I ſay the beginning, from whence the eſſence of all natural things ariſeth. The which nature Ariſtotle in another place defineth to be the beginning ſubſtantiall and the cauſe of motion,and of the reſt thereof, in the which it is at the firſt,and not by Accidents: the explication of which definition he hath comp?ehended in eight bookes.And Ariſtotle doth rightly call Nature, the cauſe and the beginning of internall motion. Fo? thoſe things which are made by Nature, and are therefo?e called naturall, haue a certaine beginning of motion , whereby they are moued of their owne acco?d, not by fo?ce. Whereby plainly appeareth the difference betwæne thoſe things which are naturall, and which

Metaph 5.
Cap.1.

C   are

are endued with an effectuall fpirit, and with power to worke by it felfe : and thofe things which are made by Arte, which haue no force nor power of doing, but are dead, and deuoided of all fenfe and motion.

By thefe things it appeareth, that things natural are called properly naturall exiftences or beings, and fuch as haue nature. And they are faide to haue nature, which poffeffe in them-felues the beginning of their motion, and of their reft : the which beginning of motion of euery thing, is either the forme or the matter, wherof we haue fpoken. Forme, which is whol-ly fpirituall, hath all her motion likewife fpirituall. So the foule is of this fame nature in a liuing creature, the motions and fences plainely celeftiall, fpirituall, and a light beginning. Whereas the Matter is terreftriall, ponderous, and corporal, the other beginning of naturall motion. By whofe waight and groffeneffe, the body tendeth downeward, fo as this kind of motion procedeth not from the foule, or fpirituall forme, but from the corporall matter, which is terreftriall and heauy by his owne nature. Hereof it commeth, that the name of nature, is giuen as well to Matter as to Forme : but more aptly and conueniently to Forme: becaufe Forme doth manifeftly giue to a thing his being, actually: whereas Matter alone can-not performe that.

For not euery liuing creature, hath fenfe and motion from that body which is folid, terreftriall and ponderous : but onely from the fpirituall forme: that is to fay, the foule mouing the body, and informing it with the vitall vertues. As for example.

A horfe is in act, and in truth a horfe, when he neither mo-ueth, leapeth, nor runneth : but thefe motions which are fpiri-tual, are the effects & operations of the foule or forme, where-as otherwife the body hauing nothing but the lineaments, and vifible forme, whereby it feemeth a horfe is meere terreftriall, heauie and deade. Howbeit, neither the foule alone of the horfe, can bee faide to bee a horfe, except it be coupled with the body.

Chymicall phyficke.

For both being ioyned and coupled together make a horfe.

Knowe therefore that the Forme is far more noble and excellent then the Matter: and that Nature as touching her effects and operations, is of that power, that it generateth, and giueth being to all things, it putteth matter on the formes, it beautifieth, and fuffereth nothing to bee corrupted, but preferueth all things in their eftate. Thefe her vertues, faculties and powers, fhe very apparantly fheweth, when as fhe worketh and caufeth all forts of beings out of the Clements, and out of the feedes and beginning of all things, Salt, Sulphur, and Mercurie: and informeth with great varietie of impreffions of the vitall fpirits, colours and tafte, and with the properties of fuch kinde of powers and faculties, that it giueth to euery thing fo much as concerneth the office and dignitie thereof, in all fufficiencie. The which building and frame of things, fo aptly and conueniently formed, in order, in number, and meafure, wee may well call diuine, not terreftriall and corporall, albeit the fame be naturall, according to the power which God hath giuen vnto Nature.

And yet wee muft not thinke that God hath fo forfaken the frame of this world, that he fitteth idle, as hauing giuen fuch admirable and potent effects to nature onely, according to the opinion of Anaxagoras, Protagoras, and many other Atheifticall Philofophers, which acknowledge no other God but Nature, as alfo did the Epicures. Who if they be fo be accufed and condemned for fo wicked an opinion, then do they deferue no fmall reprehenfion, which denie nature her partes and offices in working.

For the offices peculiar, both of her firft and fecond caufe, are to be attributed to either, according to Gods predeftination. Neither are thefe places of Scripture any thing repugnant. It is God which worketh all in all. And againe: In him wee liue, moue, and haue our beeing. For albeit this is true, yet God hath appointed Nature as a meanes to fulfill his will, the which Nature hee hauing inriched

with

with the vertues of working, he by the fame beginneth, furthereth, and perfiteth all things. Therefore the fecond caufe, is called Nature, becaufe by the fame, as by a vital inftrument, God, who is the firft caufe worketh all things. For thus God fædeth men with bread, the which he hath indued with a natural facultie of nourifhing, that the nature of bread may be faid to fæde and nourifh, whereto he hath predeftinated the fame, by the forme of natural bread.

Thus therefore thefe things are to be reconciled, that we acknowledge God to bee the firft caufe of working in all other caufes, becaufe hæ hath made the caufes, and hath giuen power of working, and doth himfelfe worke together with them, and that we beleeue that hæ ftirreth vppe, prouoketh, directeth and moderateth Nature, by the power, force, and vnitie which hæ hath giuen to her, to doe all things by her proper motions, So that we muft fæke the caufe and forme of all natural actions in Nature, which God hath made potent with fpiritual vertues, by which it acteth and worketh in the matter: for that nothing can procæde from the matter it felfe being dead, which is Vital, or indued with the faculties of working.

CHAP. IIII.

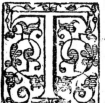

His word (Beginning) extendeth very farre. For as Artes and Sciences, fo alfo all other things haue their proper and fit beginnings. Plato intreating of Beginnings, one while appointeth three: namely, God, Patterne, and Matter: another while he appointeth two onely, that is to fay, that which is infinite, and that which is terminable, and to be limited. By the word Infinite, he meaneth Matter: and by the word Terminable, he meaneth Forme, as bringing a thing within a certaine compaffe, and reftraining a matter excurrent within bondes and limits.

Ariftotle

Ariſtotle varyed not much from the opinion and ſentence of his Maiſter, albeit he declared the ſame in other wordes, calling that Forme which Plato named Terminable. And that which Plato called Infinite; Ariſtotle nameth, Matter: appointing Priuation, by it ſelfe, for a third beginning.

Let it not therefore ſeeme abſurde to any, that we appoint three beginnings of all things, Salt, Sulphur, and Mercurie, as if it were thereby intended to ouerthrowe, by our conſtitution, the beginnings of the ancient Phyloſophers, whereas we ioyne and agrée with them. For if wée grant to Ariſtotle, his beginnings, what difference will there be betwéene him and vs. Wée admit (if you pleaſe) the diſtinction, by which he diuideth his beginnings, namely, into the firſt matter, into the ſimple matter, and into that which is remote, enduring all alterations of formes, or wherein there is power to bée made ſubiect to all formes, and in two contraryes, to wit, Forme, and Priuation: the which habilitie of taking forme, is in the ſubiect.

Wée graunt that theſe beginnings, of all other, are the more parciptible in vnderſtanding than in ſenſe. As therefore our beginnings, which we appoint out of which al mixt things are compounded and be, cannot by the Ariſtotelian Philoſophers be ouerthrowen: ſo in like Ariſtotelian beginnings cannot by ours, be deſtroyed. For all this whole world is diuided into two Globes, to wit, into the inferior Heauen, which is Aetheriall, and Aire: and into the inferior Globe, which comprehendeth Water and Earth. The ſuperior, which is Aetheriall hath in it Fire, lightning, and brightneſſe: and this firery Heauen, is a formall and eſſentiall Element.

What things ſoeuer are comprehended in theſe foure bodyes, which are the Elements and receptacles of all things, are eyther ſimple things, or bodyes, mixed and compounded of them.

They are ſimple which are without mixture, exiſting a-

C 3   part

part and seuerall by themselues : of the which all things are
made, and into the which all things are resolued. They are
compound oz corpozeat, which both are made of simples, and
into simples.

And simples may be distinguished into those things which
are simple foꝛmes, and into those which are simple matters :
oꝛ into those things which are simply foꝛmals, and into those
which are simply materials. So bodyes are diuided into materiall bodyes, and into bodyes foꝛmall.

Those things which are simply foꝛmall are astrall and
spirituall : the Elements are foꝛmall : Seedes are foꝛmall: and
the thꝛee beginnings are foꝛmall: that is to say, so spirituall, that they come not within the compasse of our sences.

But the foꝛmal Elements (whereof we speake) are they
in whose closet the astrall seedes of things, and the foꝛmal beginnings, are defused and layd vp, as in their proper receptacles : in the which simple and spirituall Elements of seedes,
and spirituall beginnings, the fruitful and quickening Sciences, properties, and rootes of propagating and increase
of al things, lye hid, wherein also all habites, dispositions,
and figures, qualities, quantities and dimentions, sauours,
odours and coolours are included, which doe budde foꝛth and
floꝛish out of their bosome in their due time, by opoꝛtune maturitie. And these simple Elements oꝛ beginnings, doe imbꝛace the spirituall seedes, with so great simphathy and friendship, and doe render to the Elements and beginnings, mutual recipꝛocation of loue, that being bꝛought by the parents, into some particular kinde, oꝛ foꝛme, they neuer make an ende,
(by the recoꝛdation of their vnion with the simple Elements)
but that at the last againe, the pꝛedestination and lithurgie of
the natural bodies being consummated, they returne backe a-
gaine to their graundfathers, and great graundfathers, and
doe rest there: euen as the floods passing and issuing out of
their Element of the sea, ꝗ running in their course hither and
thither, leauing at the length euery where behinde them their
generation (oꝛ their wombe exonerated) they returne to their
beginning

Chymicall Physicke.

beginning againe: wherupon by mutuall copulation they receiue new force and strength to increase their issue.

And this is the perpetuall circulation, by which the heauen
is marryed to the Earth, and the inferior Elements doe conioyne with the superior. For the continuall vapours arising
from the center of the earth, being expulsed into waters, and
being caryed from waters into ayre, by the attraction of the
Cœlestiall Starres: and also by the force and appetite of the
inferior Elements to bring forth issue, and to conceiue from
heauen, the sædes passing too and againe, at the last the Elements returne to their parents full and impregnated with Cœlestiall formes, and doe there nourish their sædes, vntill at the
length they bring forth in due season, and doe excluse
their generation. The which impregnation commeth
from no other, than from those astrall sædes, and these
three seuerall beginnings, Mercurie, Sulphur, and Salt,
furnished and fulfilled with all science, properties, vertues, and tinctures; and doe borrowe and fitte to themselues, out of their spirituall body, a materiall, and des
animate and adorne it with their properties. For it belongeth vnto Mercurie to giue life vnto the partes: to
Sulphur, to giue increase of body: and to Salt, to
compact those two together, and to conioyne them into
one firme body.

GOD the Creator of all things, made the world after
his owne Image, which may plainely appeare in this, that
albeit the whole world is one, yet it ioyeth in the number of
three, being framed in order, number, and measure, in whose
bosome these three simple bodyes were included, Salt, Sulphur, and Mercurie.

Therefore let vs compare the workes of God a little
with the similitude of the Trinitie. The worlde is diuided into these three partes, Intellectuall, Cœlestiall, and
Elementall. The Elementall (to let the other two alone, as
lesse knowon vnto vs) consisteth of Minerals, Vegetables, and
animals: beside the which, there is nothing to bée found in
this

this world. Of Minerals, there are thꝛee differences, Stones, Metals, and meane Minerals. In like maner among Uegitables, there are thꝛee ſoꝛts : Herbes, Trees, and Plants,

Alſo of Animals there are twꝛe oꝛders, creeping things, ſwimming things, and flying things. If we ſhould pꝛoſecute euery particular at large, wee ſhall finde this Teruarie euery where and in all the parts thereof. But we will conſider of man onely in this point.

Man conſiſteth of Spirit, Soule, and body : as holy WWꝛit teſtifieth. The Spirit ſaith, Hermes is repꝛeſented by Mercurie : the Soule is repꝛeſented by Sulphur : and the Body, by Salt. The Spirit conſiſteth of minde, reaſon, and phantaſie. The Soule hath thꝛee faculties, naturall, vitall and Animall. The Body is cut into thꝛee partes in Anatomie : to wit, into head, belly, and members. Theſe haue thꝛee pꝛincipall members, wherunto others are ſubiect : the bꝛaine, the heart, and the lyuer. The bꝛaine hath thꝛee helpes to purge by, the mouth, the noſtrils, and the eares. The purgers and receiuers of vncleanneſſe from the heart, are, the Midꝛyfe, the Lungs, and the great Arteries. The purgers of the Lyuer, are the Milt, the bladder of the Gaule, and the Reines. So there are thꝛee pꝛincipall veſſels which doe ſerue the whole body, namely, the Arteries, the Sinewes, and the Ueines. Further if we conſider the head againe, it hath thꝛee ſkinnes. The bꝛaine hath thꝛee bellyes, two ſoft befoꝛe, and one hard behinde. There are thꝛee pꝛincipall inſtruments of voyce, the thꝛoate, the pallate, and the kernels. To conclude this point, if all theſe ſhould bee diſſeuered and ſeparated into their beginnings, they might be reſolued into Mercurie, Sulphur, and Salt, whereof they conſiſt.

Therefoꝛe theſe thꝛee foꝛmall beginnings, which we haue deſcribed by their offices and pꝛopertions, albeit they are moꝛe ſpirituall than coꝛpoꝛall, yet being ioyned with ſimple Elements, they make a materiall body mixt and compound, they increaſe and nouriſh it, and pꝛeſerue it in his eſtate vnto the pꝛedeſtinated ende.

1.Theſ.5.
23.
Heb.4.12.

And

And ſeeing the properties, Impreſſions, and facultiles are inſet and incluoed in thoſe beginnings, and haue theſe vitall qualities of taſtes, odours, and colours hidden in them, how materiall ſoeuer thoſe ſeedes be: yet notwithſtanding they rather contende to come neere to Forme, than to Matter: but the Elements doe moꝛe cleaue and inclyne to Matter than to Forme. And therefoꝛe the Phyloſophers call them propeꝛly ſimple beginnings foꝛmall, becauſe they are moꝛe pꝛincipall, adoꝛned and inriched with the firſt and chiefe faculties of aſtral ſeedes. But the Elements, they call beginnings, materiall ſimple. To the one, they attribute actuall qualities, and to the other paſſiue. And ſo of them both, as it were ſeconda- rily and ſo neere as may be, all mixt bodyes are compounded and doe conſiſt.

If therefoꝛe we ſhall thꝛoughly diſcuſſe and ranſacke e- uery particular indiuidiall in his kinde, and their generation, we ſhall finde that which is ſaid to be true: namely, that ſome ſimple beginnings are foꝛmall and ſpirituall: others materiall, coꝛpoꝛall, and viſible. And that the Inuiſibles are the Elements ſimple, foꝛmall, the aſtral ſeedes, and ſpirituall beginnings. Alſo that the viſibles are all one and the ſame, but yet couered with a materiall body. The which two bo- dyes, ſpirituall and material, inuiſible and viſible, are contai- ned in euery Indiuiduall, albeit, that which is ſpirituall, cannot be diſcerned, but by reaſon of motion of life, and of functions, and yet is within it.

Theſe viſible and material bodyes are of thꝛee ſoꝛtes. $\left\{\begin{array}{l}\text{Seedes.}\\\text{Beginnings.}\\\text{Elements.}\end{array}\right.$

Of theſe 3. ſome are $\left\{\begin{array}{l}\text{Actiue, as Seeds, and Beginnings.}\\\text{Paſsiue, as are the Elements.}\end{array}\right.$

The Actiue bodies of viſi- ble Seeds, wherein there is any vertue, are $\left\{\begin{array}{l}\text{The ſeedes of liuing creatures,}\\\text{put foꝛth by Venus.}\\\text{The ſeedes of herbes \& trees, in}\\\text{their ſeueral caſes \& trunkes.}\\\text{The ſeeds of Mines, ouerwhel-}\\\text{med w a great heape of impedi-}\\\text{ments.} \qquad \text{D} \qquad \text{All}\end{array}\right.$

All which lye hidden in themfelues haue Spirits.

The Actiue bodies of
beginnings,   haue
{ Two moyſt, { Mercurie,
{   { Sulphur.
{ One dzie: Salt.

Mercurie is a ſharpe liquoz paſſable, and penetrable, and a
moſt pure ꝗ Æthereall ſubſtantiall body : a ſubſtance agile,
moſt ſubtill, quickning, and ful of Spirit, the fœde of life, and
the Eſſence, oz ſezme, the next inſtrument.

Sulphur is that moyſt, ſweat, oyly, clammy, oziginal, which
giueth ſubſtance to it ſelfe : the nouriſhment of fire, oz of natural heat, endued with the ſozce of mollifying, and of gluing
together.

Salt, is that dzy body, ſaltiſh, méerely earthſby, repzeſen-
ting the nature of Salt, endued with wonderfull vertues of
diſſoluing congealing, clenſing, emptying, and with other infinite faculties, which it exerciſeth in the Indiuiduals, and ſeperated in other bodyes, from their indiuiduals.

Theſe thzée beginnings, were by Hermes the moſt ancient Philoſopher, called Spirit, Soule, and Body. Mercurie
the Spirit, Sulphur the Soule, Salt ꝑ Body, as is already ſaid.

The body is ioyned with the ſpirit, by the bond of Sulphur : the ſoule, foz that it hath affinitie with both the extreames, as a meane coupling them together. Foz Mercury
is liquid, thinne, flexible. Sulphur is a ſoft oyle paſſable; ſalt
is dzy, thicke, and ſtable. The which netwithſtanding are ſo
pzopoztionate together, oz tempered equally the one with the
other, that a manifeſt ſigne, and great analogie oz conuenience
is found in this contrarietie of beginnings. Foz Sulphur, oz
that oyly moyſture, is as I haue ſaid) a meane, which with
his humidity, ſoftneſſe, and fl ꝗ ity oz paſſablenes, ioyneth the
two extreames, that is to ſay fixed ſalt, and flying Mercurie:
that is to ſay, the dzynes of ſalt, and the moyſtnes of Mercurie, with his viſcus and clammy humiditie: the thickneſſe
of ſalt, and the ſubtiltie of Mercurie (vtterly contary) with
his fluiditie : which holdeth the meane betwéene ſtable, and
dying. Mozeouer Sulphur, by reaſon of his exceeding ſweet-
neſſe,

neſſe, doth contemper the ſharpneſſe oʒ ſowerneſſe of Mercurie, and the bitterneſſe of ſalt : and by his clammynes, doth
contayne the ſubtill flying of Mercurie, with the firmneſſe
and faſtneſſe of ſalt.

CHAP. V.

Concerning Salt.

Ꝼ all other, the Philoſophicall ſalt is
of greateſt vertue and foʒce to purge,
and is as it were the generall clenſer of
whole nature, deliuering the ſame frem
al impuritie; whether it bee the belly, by
ſiege; the ſtomacke, by vomit; the reines,
by vrine; oʒ the body, by ſweate; ope-
ning ⁊ clenſing obſtructions, comming of what cauſe ſoeuer.

This kinde of purging is very large : whoſe partes albeit
they tend to one end, yet they haue as it were diuers ⁊ contrary effects, pʒoceeding frō one ſubiect which cannot be ſeen. And
as the effects are diuers, ſo are there diuers kindes of Saltes,
which accoʒding to their diuerſitie, haue diuers taſtes and ſun-
dery pʒoperties of euacuations and clenſings, and diuers o-
ther faculties.

But among Salts, that which is moʒe bitter and neereſt
to the taſte of Aloes oʒ Gaule, ſheweth his pʒoper woʒking in
purging the belly by ſiege. Such Salts Chymiſts call Salt-
Niter, oʒ Niterous ſalts. Saladine, an ancient ⁊ great Phyſition, ſpeaking of Salts, ſaith thus : There are foure famous
kinds of Salt, to wit, the ſalt of bread, that is to ſay Com-
mon-ſalt, ſalt-gem, ſalt-naptic, and ſalt-Indi . And afterward he ſaith, that this laſt is of all other the meſt bitter,
ſharpe, and meſt violent, and therefoʒe of greateſt foʒce to
purge. And he ſaith, that al Salt is as it were a ſpurre to o-
ther medicines with the which it is mingled : foʒ that it maketh them to woʒke moʒe ſpeedily. Laſtly, hee ſaith , that all
Salt, bʒingeth foʒth groſſe Phlegmaticke humoʒs.

Among Salts, ſome are earthie, ſome watery, and ſome

aierie,

aierie, oz such as haue in them predominant, epther the Element of that earth, of water, oz of ayze: insomuch some of
them are fixed, & are of the nature of earth: other some are betwéene fixed & flying, and doe retaine a certaine middle watery propertie. But Sal Armoniac is of nature spirituall, (as is
also the common Armoniac) & of all other most flying & ayzie.

And al Salt, whether it be flying, oz fixed, is no otherwise
dissolued and commixed in waters, than with the water of
Water, and if one be a dzy water, the other is moyst.

These thzée kindes of Saltes, which lye hydden in the secret parts of thinge, whether they be metalline, begitable, oz a-
nimal, and which are principally seated in that element, which
produceth his generations out of the earth, they do participat
of the nature of the thzée beginnings. Foz the common salte,
and that which is of the sea, passing thzough the philter of the
earth, and boyled and digested with the heates of the bowels
of the same earth, doth participate of the nature of fixed and
firme salt, the father and originall of all others. But Niter,
being partly fixed, and in part volatile, both participate of the
sulphurus beginning of things: euen as Sal Amoniac doth
participate of the Mercuriall beginning spirituall and ayzie:
whose extreames, to wit, fixed and volatile, of the sulphurus
salt, oz the Niterus, partaker of the bolatile nature in part,
and partly fixed, are coupled together by intercession. By this
straight and wonderfull bond of the thzée beginnings thzée diuers substances of Salts, of sundzy properties, doe manifestly
appeare, like in essence, but not in natures of qualities. Foz
beyond all expectation, a good wittie Salt-maker, wil extract
out of a fat and fertile earth, (by washings) these thzée kindes
of Saltes: namely, the marine and fixed, which is dissolued
in lye made of ashes, the Niterus by it selfe, which is there
coagulated oz congealed: and the Armoniac volatile & ayzie,
flying in part out of the Lye, and partly contained in both the
Saltes, and therefoze hydden from the sences. This may bée
done by a skilfull Salt-maker, albeit he were vtterly ignozant
of all the mysteries which here are hidden.

Which

Chymicall Physicke.

Which thrée distinct differences of Saltes, as they are to be found in euery fat kind of earth, so out of both the saltes, namely the marine and fired, and the Niterus volatile, they may be thenceforth separated. For those Saltes, being put into a retort together, or apart by themselues, with a receiuer, first by the force of fire stilleth forth a Volatile Salt, sower, sharpe and Mercurial: then, with a greater heate, commeth forth a Salt Sulphurus and Niterus, and swéete: the third Salt, which is Salt vpon Salt fired, will not moue with any force of fier, but remaineth constantly in the bottome of the glasse.

All tastes are brought forth out of these thrée sundry Saltes, common to that triple beginning of things, so as we shall not néede to haue recourse to hot and cold, moist and dry. For they are procreated out of those beginnings alone. Fired Salt, consider as it is simple, and without commixtion, maketh simply a salt tast. A Sulphurus Salt also simply vnderstoode, yéeldeth out of it a swéete oylely taste. But Mercurial Salt, in like sort conceiued by it selfe and apart, representeth a sower taste. All which tastes mixed together in equall proportions, yéelde a pleasant and delightful taste, without any sense or taste of any of the particulers.

These thrée beginnings cannot be found simple in a mixt body, in such wise, but that they haue some composition, and do in mixture communicate their qualities together: as may bée séene in sea-salt, and salt-péeter, out of the which may be separated not onely a salt and sharpe taste, but also a swéete taste. And it is certaine, that in things sulphurus and oylely, and also in Mercurial liquors, there is to be found a coniunction of such tastes.

For this cause we affirme, that all fired Salt of a mixt body, is very brinish and exceeding bitter: the sulphurus, of a fat and swéete taste: and the Mercurial, sower, sharpe and fiery. So that vpon these simple qualities, salt, swéete, and sower, (which are to be found in all bodies minerall, vegitable and animal) all others tastes do depend.

And as touching the elementary qualities passiue, which are

are as oꝛganical and inſtrumentall cauſes, they little apper-
taine to this matter: whether it be the terreſtrial and dꝛie paſſiue quality, & paſſiue coldneſſe, oꝛ whether it be the aierp moiſt
vapoꝛ, the which taſtes of this ſoꝛt, oꝛ potent qualities, pꝛoceedeth from theſe thꝛæ beginnings, to either further to this oꝛ
that nature, oꝛ elſe doe impaire and weaken them. To make
this plaine by manifeſt reaſons, and to lay it open befoꝛe our
eyes, we will begin to intreat of mixed bodies, the which notwithſtanding accoꝛding to the Elements, are moſt ſimple.

CHAP. VI.

T is already ſaid, that taſtes by a certaine
pꝛiuate right are aſcribed to Salts, oꝛ to
their ſpirits: which euidently appeareth
hereby, that the differences of taſtes, are
not pꝛoduced but from the differences of
Saltes: oꝛ contrariwiſe, the differences of
Salts, are pꝛoduced from the differences
of taſtes.

In the boſome of nature, there are found almoſt ſo many
kinde of Saltes, as there are variety of taſtes. Digged oꝛ minerall, and marine Salt, is endued with a ſalt qualitie. Niter with a bitter quality: Allum, with a ſharpe: Vitriol, with
a ſower: Armoniac, with a ſharpe and ſower quality. But
ſwæte Saltes do manifeſtly appeare, not onely in Manna,
and in Sugar, but alſo in marine ſalt, and in ſalt of Vitriol, out
of which they are to be ſeperated. And (as we haue ſaid) in e-
uery of theſe ſalts, theſe thꝛæ firſt beginnings, Salt, Sulphur,
and Merucry, are contained ioyntly together: one aiery, mercurial, oꝛ ſpiritual, the which is ſharpe and ſower; the other
earthly, which is ſower, and bitter: and the third oylely & ſwæt,
which is a meane betwæne them both. In Vitriol alone, is
manifeſtly to be ſæne, egar, ſharpe, ſower, and aſtringent, ſoꝛ
that of all other Salts, it is moſt coꝛpoꝛal.

But thoſe taſtes oꝛ qualities, which are mixed with paſſiue

and

and Elementarie qualities, haue not the full force of euery
of these, but are made more weake by mixtion : for the sharpe
(which is not extracted and seperated but by the force of the
fier with the aiery part) is mixed with a mercurial liquor:
the sower is mixed with a flegmatique, or watery humour:
and the eger, with a terrestrial dunouie : the which, the more
they haue of the Elementary qualities, and the same passiue,
so much the more weake they are and impaired. But if the
actiue qualities be separated from the passiue, as by arte it is to
be done, then the tarte and sower do obtaine their full force,
and doe manifestly and fully burne the tongue with their fiers:
for the sharpe hath a more fiery and burning qualitie : and the
sower, a more watery propertie. For the sharpe partaking of
the nature of fire, hath ouermuch vertue to attenuate, diffipate,
and to fret: the sower, as, aiery, watery, & of thinne parts, hath
vertue to cutte, to open, to refrigerate, and also to put away
putrifactions. The eger and more tarte, which remaineth in
the Colchotar (after the extraction of the sharpe onlely, and
sower water, with the aiery parts of the elemental qualities)
do possesse a nature and force to thicken and binde, by reason
of the earthy and grosse propertie.

But if from that terrestrial parte, the pure (which is Salt)
be extracted, it wil haue a salt taste, by the vertue whereof it
wil bee made, both deiectiue, and vomitiue. And in the sweete
Sulphur of Uitriol, there is a manifest sweetnesse, which is
plainely stupefactiue.

Finally, in all Salts, almost, (discouered by Chymicall seperation) these three are to be discerned, Sower, Sweete, and
Bitter, which haue force of actiue qualities, and yet not destitute of the moist passiue, terrestrial and grosse, but with them,
in sundry wise so seasoned and tempered, that they bring to the
Salts, varety of tastes.

And let this serue for demonstration, by which it may
plainely appeare, that those sundry differences of tastes, are
manifestly contained in Salts, both ioyntly and seuerally,

especially

efpecially in their fpirits : And accoꝛding to the opinion of Hermes fchollers, we deny that thofe infet and naturall qualities, vertues, and pꝛoperties, are to be arrogated to hotte, moiſt, and dꝛie, but rather to the eſſences of a nature which is falt, bitter, eger, fharpe, fower, tarte, fwéete, and oylely.

Foꝛ there are fire hundꝛed frigidities oꝛ coldes, fire hundꝛed heates, humidities, & figities oꝛ dꝛineſſes, then the which nothing doth moꝛe heate, cœle, moyſten, and dꝛy. But they haue neuer bꝛought any fauour oꝛ taſte to pure oꝛ fimple water, oꝛ to other Iuices oꝛ liquoꝛs, which haue béene deſtitute of Salt.

Whatfoeuer is without Salt, oꝛ deſtitute of a bꝛiniſh fpirit, can neuer be diſcerned by taſte, but is vtterly vnfauoꝛy. Yet notwithſtanding, if fimple water be powꝛed vpon aſhes, with a little heate, that water wil dꝛawe vnto it faltneſſe, bitterneſſe, oꝛ fharpneſſe, moꝛe oꝛ leſſe, accoꝛding to the nature of the falt, moꝛe oꝛ leſſe falt, oꝛ bitter, which is contained in the aſhes.

And if any man obiect, that Hony and Sugar by boyling, oꝛ by the foꝛce of fier, may be made fharpe oꝛ bitter: we anſwer that it commeth fo to paſſe, when the aiery fulphurus, and watery partes, which bꝛing and pꝛeferue the fwéetneſſe do periſh and are feparated by decoction. But terreſtrial Salt, whofe faculties are inward, haue this pꝛoperty, that of their owne nature they poſſeſſe, this oꝛ that fharpe oꝛ bitter taſte, how extreame foeuer it be. So if thou ſhalt dꝛawe out of onions and garlicke a Volatile and aiery fharpe Mercurial Salt, which ariſeth in the fuperficies & vppermoſt of their bodies: thou ſhalt make them moꝛe fwéet and pleafing, and to put off their fharpneſſe, by which they bite the tongue: but yet they will retaine and repꝛefent their hot qualitie, with the which they abound, by reafon of their fixed Saltes. As out of Saltes, fo out of odours alfo, we may dꝛawe certaine faculties, without the helpe of hotte qualities. Foꝛ féeing they are referred to the diuers pꝛoperties of Sulphur, fundꝛy odours dos arife therfrom, and not from the qualities. Which if they be fwéete and pleafing, the

bꝛaine

bʒaine receiueth them with pleaſure and delight, whereas vnpleaſant ſauours oʒ odours, are offenſiue both to the noſe and to the bʒaine, and are reiected. Such is the narcotical and ſtefactiue odour of Poppie, and Hemlock, and ſuch like which do ſtinke, and aſtoniſh the bʒaine, by reaſon (as Phyſitions affirme) of their colde qualitie: Wherein they bʒeake the Lawe of their axiomes, foʒ that they holde that their odours are of a hotte qualitie, as moſt true it is. Foʒ that which is ſtupefactiue in the Poppeis, and in Opium, is no other thing, but a certaine oylely and ſulphurus parte conceiuing flame, (much like to that kinde of oyle, which is extracted out of the ſeedes of Poppey) the which albeit it do readily burne, yet as it is commonly thought, it ſhe weth moſt colde effects. The common Phyſitians, to coʒrect ſuch coldneſſe attributed to Opium, vſe helpes, as is to bee ſeene in their opiat and antidotarie medicines, wherin Opium is an Ingredient. Of theſe kind of cõpoſitions Myrepſus deſcribeth aboue foure ſcoʒe: where Euphorbium (which is of a fiery and burning facultie) is no moʒe foʒboʒne then either of the Peppers, oʒ ſuch other like cauſticke and burning ſimples, of extreame hotte qualitie: when as the true and pʒoper coʒrectoʒ of Opium (that I may ſo ſpeake) wel knowne to Hermeticall Phyſitians, is Vineger; which putteth away ſtupefactiue vapours and fumes, that they aſcende not to the bʒaine, ſo ſuppʒeſſing them by the ſharpneſſe thereof, that it retaineth them: whereas their hot coʒrectoʒs do moʒe ſtirre them vp and multiple them. Hereof come ſiniſter and deadly paſſions and paines, by reaſon whereof men are conſtrained to vſe the imperfect Laudanum of Empiricks, againſt the deadly daunger of ſuch medicines.

CHAP.

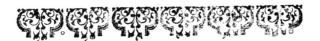

CHAP. VII.

Ow fomewhat fhall be faide concerning colcurs. The dogmatical Phyfitians, that they might not diminifh any whit of the qualities of colours; are wont to referre to thofe qualities a certaine varie- y of colours: and haue obferued and no- ed certaine friuolous and light obferuati- ons: as when they fay, that in a white onion, oz in white wine, a man may iudge by the colour a great coldneffe, than in a read onion, oz in red wine. Whereas white fublimate, and Arfnic, albeit they are moft white like vnto Chziftall: yet neuertheleffe vnder this whiteneffe, they fofter and hide a moft burning and deadly fire. Yea Sugar it felte, which is fo fwæt, white, and pleafant, doth hide in the innermoft parts thereof, a wonderfull blackneffe and fharpneffe, from whence may bée extracted moft fharpe liquozs and waters, which will dif- folue and bzeake the moft hard metalls. Therefoze it is ab- furd, to fharpe and fozme colours from hotte and colde, which do pzocæde from the fpirits only, oz elfe trom the moft thinne and aiery bapozes, which lye hid in the Salt: efpecially in that Salt which by nature is fulpharus, fuch as is Niter, oz Salt- Peter, as men call it. Niter thzoughly depured and clenfed, will be as white as fnow; from which whiteneffe, may be dzawen infinite fozts of colours, moft excellent to beholde. Which colours come from the onely fpirits of Salt-peter, which are able to pearce the moft hard kind of glaffe, by the fozce of fire thzuft fozth in the likeneffe of volatile meale, and cleauing in the ouerture of the glaffe Alembic. By which co- lours, a mã may behold the body of the Alembic to be tained & dyed, as well within as without in the fuperficial part: Which colours are of no leffe varietie, then are the flowers of the earth in the time of the Spzing. Hereby it appeareth plainely, that this diuerfitie of all colours is to be taken trom the fpirits,

no leſſe noʒ otherwiſe, then are all other pʒoperties and vertues of all other things to be referred vnto them.

If therefoʒe the foundation of theſe thʒœ things be laid vpon thʒœ beginnings, & vpon their ſpirits, it will be very ſirme
and ſtable, in ſuch wiſe, that in the ignoʒance of any cauſe, it
ſhal not be nœdful to ſlye to hidden pʒoperties.

If this doctrine, accoʒding to the truth thereof, be receiued, learned, and ſtudied, being vpholden alſo with the autho-
rities of that great Hypocrates, it ſhal eaſily dʒiue from vs
the darkeneſſe of ignoʒance, and ſhal bʒing with it the light of
knowledge, which will remoue all difficulties : Foʒ out of
this ſchœle are learned moſt certain and infallible Thearemes
and Axiomes, againſt which, as againſt moſt aſſured grounds,
there can be no oppoſition oʒ reſiſtance : but wil be allowed by
the general conſent of indifferent Judges.

Let vs take an example from Vineger : whereof many famous Phyſitians cannot tell what certainely to affirme. Foʒ,
becauſe it is ſharpe, and therefoʒe cœleth, they wil haue it to
be colde. But contrariwiſe, when they behold the facultie
thereof, to be attenuating, cutting, and diſſoluing, alſo their
fernoʒ and boyling thereof, when it is put vpon earth oʒ claie,
they are conſtrained to foʒſake their opinion, vncertaine what
to iudge thereof. Who, if they had bene acquainted with
the Hermeticall doctrine, they ſhould haue knowne, that the
cauſe of ſuch tartneſſe oʒ ſowerneſſe in vineger, commeth by
the ſeperation of the ſpirit, from the wine: as is plainly ſœne by
experience. Foʒ the longer that wine ſtandeth in the Sun, oʒ
in a hotte place, the moʒe by little and little it wareth ſharpe;
and whatſoeuer is aiery therein, and of the quinteſſence of the
wine, by the foʒce of the heat vapoʒeth away This eternal and
celeſtial eſſence being gone, which was the cauſe of the wines
ſwœtnes (which ſwœtnes hath alwaies ioyned with it neuertheleſſe, a certaine pʒicking very acceptable to the pallate, by
reaſon of a ſingular temper of ſharpneſſe Vitriolated by
ſwœte and Sulphurus ſpirits, put by the inſtinct of nature
into wine) at the length it wareth ſower : the cauſe of
whoſe ſharpneſſe, is not to be referred to the colde qualities,

but

but to thofe hidden and fower fpirits of Salt, which by the bonde of the fulphurus fubſtance, were contained and kept in their office and woꝛking in the wine : the which bond being diſſolued, the fpirits range at will, and doe make manifeſt their nature, which was afoꝛe hidden. Hereupon it commeth, that vnegers are ſharper in one foꝛt, then in another, accoꝛding as they haue in them moꝛe oꝛ leſſe of the nature of Salt Armoniac, and no whit of the fulphurus fubſtance. Foꝛ ſimple water deuoide of all Salt, can neuer by reaſon of the coldneſſe therein waxe fower. But as from wine, fo from meat, and from ale oꝛ béere, and from boyling new wine, may be feparated the pꝛoper water of life, and ethereal fubſtance, the which being fo feparated, they become eager, becaufe they containe in themfelues a ſharpe falt of nature.

Such is that ſharpe falt, which Phylofophers call their Mercury, oꝛ Salt Armoniac, Uolatile and fpiritual (becaufe of al metalline falts, the common Armoniac is moſt Uolatile, ſuch as in the foꝛme of moſt white and falt meale, may be carried vp vnto the cloudes by fublimation, and yet hath a dꝛy and fpiritual nature, which the Phylofophers call their dꝛy water: becaufe this Salt is fo farre foꝛth Uolatile and flying, that it is lifted vp together with the aiery oꝛ watery vapour, of the which is made the mixture of the compound: and fo great is the ſharpneſſe of this falt, that one fcruple oꝛ eightéene oꝛ twenty graines of this falt perfitly refined and made moſt fimple, diſſolued in a pot of commom water, doth make all the fame wonderfully fower.

And this is the Salt, (the fulphurus eſſence taken away) which ſheweth it felfe euidently to be féene by his ſharpneſſe in vineger, with watery fubſtance. But the moꝛe ſtrong the wine ſhal be, the moꝛe ſharpe the ferment of the vineger, and the moꝛe vehement the tartneſſe thereof will ſhewe it felfe: out of the which the pearcing, attenuating, ⁊ diſſoluing fpirits, are extracted by a ſkilful woꝛkmã the which foꝛces ⁊ faculties cannot pꝛocéed from any other thing, then from that fpiritual and Uolatile falt Armoniac, mixed with a watery humour.

And

And to make this more plaine, and to proue it by effect, take the most strong Vinegar, white or red : distil the same in Balneo Mariæ, till it be drie, with a gentle fire, out of a pinte and a halfe, you shall extract thrée partes or more, like most cleare water, but most sharpe and sower, the bottome of the matter as the lées and pheses remaining in the bottome of the glasse with the most sharpe and byting Salt, the which, because it is fixed, and cleauing to the terrestrial part of the Uinegar, cannot be extracted but by the great violence of the fire. By which meane a most sharpe oyle, like in nature to Aqua Regia, most corroding and fretting, is extracted, not by reason of the heate of fire, but by the force and power of a brinish substance which is expelled in forme of an oyle with the Salt from the rest of the feces, by fire.

But leauing that sharpe fire of the Lées, let vs take in hand to explicate the sowernes of the Uineager distilled. By a soft and gentle distillation, is first of all extracted, a certaine watry elementary phleme, which is drawne out of the whole body almost without taste, leauing in the bottome of the glasse, another liquour, farre more sower and sharpe, and therefore more strong to dissolue, which otherwise before was nothing so sharp, because the Salt Armoniac was tempered and mixed with a watry Phleame. Whereof if thou desire to know the quantitie, take so much of the best Salt Tartar, which is of the same nature, but fixed, by which if thou drawe by little and little thrée pintes of this Uinegar distilled, and disphleamed, to the waight of one ounce, thou shalt finde the volatile Salt Armoniac to be conioyned with the sharpe fixed Salt : and that which shall be distilled from the same, will become altogether without taste, or a little swéetish, the volatile Salt Armoniac being gone, through the passage in the fixed Salt. So that the said ounce of Salt Tartar, is increased by one scruple or more of volatile Salt, increasing the quantitie of the other fixed. Thus that volatil Salt Armoniac which vanisheth out of the Uinegar with the watry and aierie substance is retained by passage, in the proper fixed Salt, and there abideth, and by his absence, dispoyling the distilled li-

C 3   sour,

quoz, of all fowerneffe: the which is therefoze of no vertue, oz of leffe efficacie, then pure and fimple water. Hereby it appeareth, how litle ferment is needful to a great quantitie of pafte, to acuate and augment the fame, as Phylofophers fpeak: without the which, the elementary water wil haue no fharpeneffe. Foz if that Salt Armoniac be wanting, as touching the fozce and vertue thereof, water hath neither tartneffe, noz tafte at all.

Therefoze a Hermetical Phylofopher ¢ Phifitian, which is wel acquainted with the liuely anatomie of things, wil teach, that the fharpe, fower, and attennating tafte of vineger, and the diffoluing facultie thereof, arifeth herehence, becaufe tart things, whether they be waters, oz iuices, are mixed and infufed with falt Armoniac: and that therefoze Uineger, not onely in regard of the tartneffe thereof, but alfo that moft thin fpirituous fower effence of Salt, doe pierce into the moft inward parts euen of the hard bodyes. And if it fhewe foyth any cœling effects, it commeth thereof, becaufe the fulphurus, and fierie qualitie of the wine, that is to fay, the *Aqua Vitæ*, is feperated: without the feperation whereof it can neuer bee made vineger, and can at no time yælde any tafte of *Aqua Vitæ*. And that fharpeneffe by which it burneth, is the chariot oz carrier away, of the elementarie and colde water, by the which it is carryed and pierceth into the moft inward and fecret partes, as thee haue learned by often experience, that in that water, the fame fharpneffe is contained, and moft næerely coniopned therewith.

Nowe, as we haue fhewed that the fower and mercuriall liquoz of things, doth bozrow that tartneffe, from a certaine Armoniac falt, and volatile, which arifeth from the fixed: euen fo the fulphurus and oylie liquoz, doth receiue and taketh his vertue from no other thing, than from that fwæte Biterous fulphurus falt, which bozroweth the fame from fixed falt: fo that, in the fixed falt, and out of that falt, that mercuriall fowerneffe, and fulphurus vertue doe fpzing, and

and doe receiue their fruits thereto, as from the roote and first originall.

As also héere it is to be noted, and to be wondred at, that a tryple substance is seuerally to be extracted, out of one and the same Essence: from whence all things created, do sucke and drawe their faculties, vertues and properties: and that the same doe so subsist in one and the same subiect, that two others are to be produced from one other. And the same thrée essences, when they are separated, and coupled together againe and vnited, are then inriched and increased with wonderfull vertues and faculties, and haue gotten excéeding perfection. The which, the more often that they be separated and vnited, the more perfect and high degrées of power and force they obtaine: in such wise, that it is to bée reputed the vniuersall and most excellent Medicine of all others.

CHAP. VIII.

Concerning the excellent goodnesse of Salt
in Medicine, according to
auncient prescription.

I is manifest in the Writings of Galen, and other Greeke Physitians, as also in the Traditions of the Arabians and Latines, with one consent, that Salt is good and profitable, not onely to season and sawce meates, but also for Medicine: Albeit in the dyet of sicke persons, they commanded them to abstaine from salt things: They defended the vse of Salt, to be necessary for the curing of diuers diseases, for that it hath vertue, to clense, to open, to cut, and to make thinne, to moue sweates, to further vrine, and to prouoke vomit.

And

And in this manifold facultie and vertue, it is more profitable than the most of other remedies. For the proofe whereof we will bring certaine examples of some of the most auncient and famous Physitians.

Lib.de re-
med.7.cap.3

First of all Ægineta, concerning the facultie of Salt, saith
thus: All Salt, hath great facultie to drye and to binde:
Wherefore it consumeth all whatsoeuer is moyst in mens
bodyes: and compacteth the rest by binding. For this
cause it preserueth from putrifaction. But burnt Salt hath
greater force to resolue and consume.

Lib.collec.
15.

Oribasius is of the same opinion, Saltes, (saith he) whether they be digged out of the earth, or whether they come out
of the sea, haue like facultie: and is mixed with two qualities,
that is to say, of clensing, and binding. In this notwithstanding they differ, that Saltes digged out of the earth, are of a
resoluing and consuming essence, by reason that they are of
more grosse parts, and do more binde.

Lib.2. de
virtute simp.
medi. ad
Eutrapi.

The same Oribasius, saith also, speaking of Aloes, digged and marine salt haue all one force, and are mixed of two
qualities, the one of clensing, the other of binding. But it
is plaine, that both kindes doe drie. For the which cause it
consumeth all humor in the body, and thickeneth the solyde
parts by binding. Burnt salt hath greater force to clense:
but it doth not contract and thicken so much as the other.

The flower of salt, hath thinner parts, than burnt salt, and
is of a sharpe qualitie and much digesting.

Tetr 1.
serm. 2. cap.
43. & 46.

Aetius hath also almost the same woordes: sauing that hee
addeth this concerning the froth of salt: The flower of Salt
saith hee, is frothy, cleauing to the rockes that are next adioyning, and it hath by nature more thinne partes, than Salt it
selfe, therefore it can much more attenuate and resolue: but
the rest of the substance, cannot thicken as Salt doth.

Paulus Aegineta, in the same Booke and chapter before
quoted, writeth that the same froth of Salt, is the flower of
Salt, and is of more thinne parts, and more consuming, then
is Salt it selfe, but doth lesse compact. By which it doth euidently

dently appeare, that the science of Calcination, of attenuation, and of essences, was not vnknowen to them of olde time. For by the working and styrring of the sea, they learned the Art of distillation, by which they seperated the more spirituous, from the more grosse: euen as we see the truth hereof to appeare in the experience of charming and working simple milke. For by that meanes, three sundrie substances, are diuided one from the other, namely Butter, Curdes, and Whaye.

Ætius, speaking of crudities, and of those things which do helpe concoction, according to the opinion of Galen, and other Physitians, setteth before vs Saltes: In the description whereof, he putteth in, one pound of salt of Cappadocca, the which surmounteth the dose of all other the Ingredients of that composition: the which poulored, he prescribeth to be taken in a reare egge, to the quantitie of halfe a spoonefull, fasting in the morning. The effect whereof he sheweth in these words: No man can sufficiently commende the worthines of this medicine, for the helping vertue which it hath in colde distemperatures, correcting raw humors: for the which cause it helpeth the collicke, and doth gently losen the belly.

He describeth also other saltes which losen the bellie, which drawe fleame from the head, with other helpes besides. And into one composition, hee appointeth to be put of cleere dryed salt, 144. dragmes. In the which composition, hee added of the flowers of Chamamil, of Coniza, of mountaine Calamynt, of the roote of the mountaine Eringium, of Origan, of Sylphium, of Pepper, of each a thirde parte. The which Ingredients put to the quantitie of the salt aforesaid, come nothing neere to the quantity therof.

He appointeth another composition of Salte: where to thirtie ounces of parched salt, hee appointeth a farre lesse dose of Hysope, of wilde Tyme, & of Cummine: the continuall vse whereof, hee appointeth in steede of common salte, not onely for to make the meate sauory, but also for medicine. For (saith he) who so vseth the same continually, shall at no time be troubled with any disease. It helpeth headache, it quickeneth the sight, it cleanseth the brest from fleame, it maketh good concoction in the stomacke, and purgeth the kidneys.

Ter. 3. serm.
1. cap. 24.

F   Hereby

Hereby it appeareth, that the auncient Phyſitians did not only vſe Salt, but alſo that they made choyſe of the beſt and moſt cleare ſort, the which alſo they dryed and parched with heate of the fire, to make it the more forcible to helpe in all obſtructions. For Salts are of that power, that they take away all manner putrifaction and corruption of wormes, and doe put away the originall of other vices and diſeaſes, and do amend them. The which being ſo, what other thing can be found out, for the conſeruation of life and health, or for the expulſion of all diſeaſes, more profitable.

Actuarius, alſo deſcribing certaine purgatiue Salts, doth giue In lib. de metho. me-de. cap. 9. vnto them great efficacie in helping and eaſing ſundry diſeaſes, and in preuenting many ſickneſſes.

Myrepſius deſcribeth moe then twenty ſundry Salts. And among their compoſitions, hee calleth one the Apoſtles Salt, the which preſerueth the ſight to a very great age, clenſeth the lunges from tough fleame, preuenting coughes, and inlarging the breath. Another compoſition hee attributeth to Saint Luke the Euangeliſt, which is almoſt of the like vertue, the which the Prieſtes of Aegipt, (as he ſaith) vſed for fulneſſe, that they might be the more fitte to apply themſelues to their ſtudies : being alſo of force, to remedie ſundry diſeaſes.

Marcellus Empiricus diſcribed two maner of purging Salts. Li. de medi-dica. cap. 30. Many other authors might be alleaged, as Gregorius Theologus, Plinius Secundus, and others, which haue giuen great commendation to the vertue of Salts, whoſe wordes for breuities ſake, I omit.

CHAP. IX.

Concerning the extractions of Salts out of all things, and Chymicall calcinations and incinerations, knowne to the ancient Phyſitians, and vſed in Medicine.

There

THere are some which contemne and deride our Artifice concer-ning the extractions of Salts. But no wise man will speake againſt the thing which he knoweth not. For the auncient Phyſiti-ans, haue vſed calcinations like vnto ours : as may appeare by the wordes of Oribaſius, when he maketh mention of the Calcinati-on of Tartar, and of the feces of vineger, put into an earthen potte, cloſe paſſed or luted. For he ſaith that the matter which is to be cal-cined, being faſt luted in a potte, and ſet ouer the fire to be baked, ſo long, vntill it waxe white, Alchimically.

Plinius Secundus, vſed the aſhes of beaſtes and foules, as moſt ſingular and familar remedies.

All the auncient writers, ſpeaks of a little bird like a Wrenne, which is called Regulus Troglodites, and haue taught that the ſame being brought into aſhes, is ſingular remedie for the Stone. Alſo they ſay, that glaſſe calcined and burnt into aſhes, hath the ſame effect. And many of our later Phyſitians, doe vſe the aſhes of a ſponge, drunke in white wine, for the cure of the Broncoceles, which is a diſeaſe ariſing from the throates kernells, of ſome cal-led the Hermia of the throate. This they preſcribe to be drunke for the ſpace of one whole Moone : which is a moſt certaine experience.

Aetius propoundeth many and ſundry remedies, which they of olde time vſed, which being calcined and diſſolued into aſhes, accor-ding to the common faſhion of Chymiſts, be moſt highly eſtéemed, as ſecrets of excéeding price. His wordes are theſe. It is ſaid, that if harts horne be burnt and waſhed, it cureth the diſentery Fluxe, and the ſpitting of blood : and is giuen with great profit to them that haue the Jaundiſe : being giuen in the quantitie of two ſpoonefulls. And in another place he ſaith : Some burne the clawes of Swine, and giue the aſhes to thoſe that are tormented with the collicke, in drinke. Other ſome ſay, that Aſſes houes burnt, drunke daily & doe cure the falling ſicknes. Againe he ſaith, All burnt bones haue pow-er to drie away & to dry vp : but more eſpecially mens bones. Much more might be brought out of Aetius concerning theſe things, to proue that they of olde, did vſe calcinations and aſhes, in diuers and ſundry maladies. Albeit all aſhes in generall, ſo farre forth as they containe in them their proper Salt, haue power in them to dry vp, & to clenſe, yet neuertheleſſe they retaine in them ſome property of that matter out of the which they are extracted.

Ter. 1.
Ser. 2.

Cap. 156.

Cap. 157.

Cap. 161.

F 2   And

Lib. 7. de
re medica.

And this agreeth with that which Ægineta teacheth, faying:
Afhes haue not exactly one temperature, but do differ according to
the difference of the matter which is brent. And therfore the afhes
of fharp things, as of Oakes, or Holme, do binde very much, and
do ftoppe the eruption of bloud without any other thing. But the
afhes of more fharp things, as of the figge, and Tythimal, or fpurge,
are more fharpe and cleanfing.

Coll. lib. 15.

Oribafius wryteth in like manner, fauing that he proceedeth
further. For he plainely teacheth the Chymicall extraction of falt
out of fuch afhes, fpeaking thus: Afhes (faith hee) haue in them,
partly that which is Earthie, and partly that which is fumie, and
thefe partes are thinne, and the afhes fteeped or infufed in water,
and ftrayned, do paffe through together: that which remaineth being earthie and weake, and without byting, is made hotte, hauing
put of his force in the watering or infufion. And thus Oribafius
calleth the feparation of the actiue from the paffiue & earthie (which
he calleth infirme, or weake, but the Chymifts, the deade and damned earth) Seperation.

All whatfoeuer our more fkilfull Chymifts of this age could
adde vnto the Calcinations and Jncinerations of the more ancient,
is this one thing, that out of fuch kinde of Afhes (whereof Oribafius maketh mention) they drawe out the whole water, and drye
it vp: and that which remaineth in the bottome, being impure falt,
they diffolue againe with common water, or with the proper water
thereof, (which is better) diftilled from it, before the Jncineration of
the matter, that they may make the fame cleane and pure, and as
cleere as Chryftall. For they diffolue many times, they fylter, and
coagulate, not to the vttermoft poynt of dryneffe: but drawing out
onely of that water two thirde partes and more, by the pipe of the
Alembick, they afterward remooue the fame from the fire, that the
falt therein contained, and fet in a colde place, may growe into a
chryftalline Jfe, which is the moft pure falt of the matter without
all doubt. This falt muft be gathered together, and feparated with
a woodden fpoone. And if there remaine any parte of the water, let
it bee vapoured againe, and then putte into a veffell to ftand in the
colde ayre, where will bee contealed a chryftalline refidence anew,
which

which must be seperated againe, ouer and ouer so many times, vntill moze it can growe into a Iellie oz Ise. These kinde of Ise re-
cidences, are the true beginning of Salts, vital and qualified with
admirable vertues. And this salt hath in it still the other two sub-
stantiall beginnings, Sulphur, and Mercury. Foz from the same,
the mercuriall and sulphurcous beginning, the one sweete and vnctuous, the other sharpe and Etheriall, may yet bee dzawen by a skilfull wozkeman the moze fixed parte, namely that of Salt, remaining still in the bottome. Saltes haue their cozpozall Impurities,
but the spirituall Balsam which lyeth hidde in them, is the Chymicall salte, knowen to a fewe. Some of these Salts are bytter as
wozmewood, some sweete as sugar, some sharpe as vitriolls, sower
as Quinces oz grapes, by whose balsame they are nourished, foste-
red, and conserued. These salts haue diuers spirites, some resoluing, some coniealing: And as they haue diuers spyzits, so do they
wozke sundzie and admirable effects.

<h2 style="text-align:center">CHAP. X.</h2>

Wherein is prooued, that the naturall and originall moysture in Saltes, is not consumed by calcination, but that
the very formes do lye hidde in that con-
stant and vitall beginning.

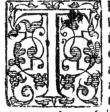He Naturall and oziginall moysture, with the
which Saltes are replenished (as is afozesaid)
is not consumed with the fozce of fire, and by
Calcination. Foz it shall be here shewed, that
all the moze fozcible tinctures and impzessions,
and the pzoperty of things, together with their
most potent qualities and powers, as tastes,
odours, colours, with the very fozmes themselues, & such like, are
concluded, and do lie hid, in that firme, constant, & vitall beginning.

Foz the truth whereof, I will deliuer vnto you certaine demon-
strations, oftentimes pzoued and confirmed by my owne experience. One, I learned of a friend which lodged at my house, who
was

was the first Inuentor therof. Another, I receiued frõ a most learned & famous Polonian, a skilfull Physitian, aboue 26. yeers since.

This man was so excellently, and phylosophically skilfull in
the preparing of the ashes out of al the parts of any maner of plant,
with all the Tinctures and Impressions of all the parts of the
plant, and would in such wise conserue all their Spirites , and
the Authours of all their faculties, that hée had aboue thirtie
such plants prepared out of their ashes of diuers sorts, conteyned in their seuerall glasses, sealed vp with Hermes seale, with
the tytle of each particular plant, and the propertie thereof, written
vpon the same. So, as that if a man desired to sée a Rose or Mary-
gold, or any other flower, as a red or white Poppey, or such like:
then would hée take the glasse wherein the ashes of such a flower
was inclosed, whether it were of a Rose, a Marie golde, a Poppey, a Gilly flower, or such like, according as the writing of the
glasse did demonstrate. And putting the flame of a Candell to the
bottome of the glasse, by which it was made hote, you might sée
that most thinne and impalpable ashes, or salt, send forth from the
bottome of the glasse, the manifest forme of a Rose, vegetating and
growing by little and little, and putting on so fully the forme of
stalkes leaues and flowers, in such perfect and naturall wise in apparant shew, that a man would haue beléeued verily, the same to
be naturally corporeat, whereas in truth it was the spirituall Idea,
indued with a spirituall essence: which serued for no other purpose,
but to be matched with his fitting earth, that so it might take vnto
it a more soly body. This shadowed Figure, so soone as the vessell
was taken from the fire, turned to his ashes againe, and banishing
away, became a Chaos and confused matter.

When I had séene this secret, & endeuouring with al my might to
attaine to the same, I spent much time about it, but yet lost my labour. But as touching the demonstration following: I affirme vpon my faith and credite, to be most certaine, and haue often proued
and experimented it by my selfe & may easily be done by any man.

The Lord de Luynes Formentieres , a man of great account, both for his learning and office , being noble , and of all men
singularly beloued , long since departed this life : with whom in
his life time, I conuersed with great familiaritie. This noble man
toolke very great paines , to search and finde out the most excellent
secrets

secrets of nature, but specially those which appertained, either for the preseruatiō, oꝛ foꝛ the restoꝛing of health. And seeking long to find such remedies, foꝛ that he had languished in a craȝed boḋy a great while without any helpe, and was iudged by Physitians to be past cure, he was at the last holpen, and wonderfully restoꝛed to health, by one only Lossenge of a certaine Chymical electuary of great vertue, which the Lady de la Hone, a most noble and wise matrone gaue vnto him. This Lossenge, prouoked him to easie vomit, by which he cast vp from his stomacke all impurity, tough and discens, like the whites of egs, diuersly coloured, in great quantitie: by which hee was restoꝛed to health againe, to his great ioy and comfoꝛt.

Hereupon he greatly desireth to know this secret, the which he not onely obtained at the hands of that noble Lady, but some others also no lesse vertuous, by his own endeuour afterwards: the which he vsed both foꝛ his owne health, & also foꝛ the good of others as need required, in the way of Chꝛistian charity. This man cōming out of France, in the time of the ciuil wars, & conuersing with me, applyed his mind to extract Salt out of mettals: that thereby he might pꝛepare a remedy against the stone, dissoluing it with cristall. This Salt being mixed with the lye made with ashes of but vꝛt meṫalꞌs, by often powꝛing warme water vpon the same, & dꝛawing it thꝛough too and againe (as women are wont to make their cōmon lye) shewed a pꝛofe of his essence, included in the lye after this maner.

The lye being strained thꝛough a Filter, & oftentimes very well clensed, was put into a bessell of earth, hauing a narrow bottom, and a wide mouth, which is called a Terime. And when the said bessell had stood without the windowes in the cold aire, by the space of one night, it grew into an Ise, thꝛough the cold of the winter. The window being opened early in the moꝛning, and the lye clensed there appeared a meere and firme Ise, wherein there appeared a thousand foꝛmes of mettalls, with all the parts thereto belonging: as leaues, stalkes, and rootes. being very plaine and apparant to the eye of the beholders, in such soꝛt as no man could but acknowledge them to be mettals.

When the noble man beheld this, and gazed vpon it, as on a miracle, he hastily ranne vnto me, and spake to me in the woꝛds of Archymides, crying, I haue found, come, and see. And when I came into his woꝛke-house, I tooke the Ise, and bꝛake of a good peece, péece, which I handeled so warily, that it might not melt with the warmth of my hand, and carryed it to men of great woorth, which dwelt with vs in that Citie: who beholding the Ile, affirmed most constantly that they were mettalls, and did no lesse maruaile then I my selfe did, wondering what it should intende, and from whence, and how so excellent a thing coulde procéede out of Nature: wée all calling to minde this sentence of holie writ: *Remember man, that thou art Ashes, and to Ashes againe thou shalt returne*: considering that the forces of such things do lye hydde and abide in their ashes, from whense the Resurrection of our Bodies is most assuredlie to bée expected.

This gallant experiment being afterwards oftentimes by mée wrought, & rightly perfoomed by Art, brought also to my minde that Historp wherof I spake before, concerning a *Poleland* Physitian: the which when I saw, I stroue, and endeuozed all that I coulde, with meditation and practice to bring it to passe. And first I thought vpon the reasons how so excellent a woorke might be finished: and what it was, that gaue foome so perfectly to a Rose, or to any other Plant, accozding to the verie life, with all the Naturall colours thereto belonging, in a moment, occasioned through a light heate. I say, I had diuers and sundzie cogitations with my selfe how this thing might bée. And amyddest these thoughts, and as I was bu-sied in other woozkes, I perceiued that the foome and figure of a thing is included in his salt, without any colour: and that there are no other colours in water, then waterie, that is to say white: And further, that the mettalls in that I sée should be deuoid of all colour, sauing waterie and white, by reason that the Ethereall and Mercu-riall spirites Uapozous and sulphurous do banish away, by their as-sation and calcination in the Sunne shine. from the which spirits the colours doe arise, as is to be séene in Salt Niter: which al beit whyte in shewe, yet put into a close Lembic, and set ouer the fire in sande to be fixed, it sendeth foozth his flying spirits, euen through the harde bodie of the Alembic, of fiue hundzeth seuerall colours, and cleauing to the vttermost part of the vessell like volatile meale. Sée-ing therefoze there lye hid so many sundzie colours in Salt-peter, (which is a fatte salt of the earth) there is no doubt but that the like

saltes

Saltes alſo are contained in all other things, which containe in them their proper colours alſo drawen out of the power of the earth, which ſhew forth themſelues in their due ſeaſon by the induſtrie of Art.

Thus after long deliberation had with my ſelfe, I fullie reſolued to make tryall hereof. And firſt I tooke one whole ſimple being in this perfect vigor and ſtrength in the ſpring time, hauing fulneſſe of Iuice, and impreſſions of vitall tinctures, which natures are includes in the ſpirites of Saltes. This ſimple (I ſay) I determined to beate in a marble morter, with his ſtalkes, leaues and flowers, together with the rootes, and ſo to reduce it into a *Chaos* or confuſed maſſe, & to put it into a veſſell of glaſſe, cloſed with Hermes ſeale, and ſo to remaine to be digeſted, macerated, and fermented a conuenient time, out of the which at the length I might extract thoſe three principles, Salt, Sulphur, and Mercurie, & to ſeparate them according to arte, preſeruing with all diligence the ſpirtes: & out of their mercuriall and ſulphurous liquor actiue, ſeparating the Elementall water paſſiue, whereby is extracted out of the drie Feces artificially calcined , a Salt, brought to the puritie of Chriſtall, which is a moſt white aſhes, and moſt full of life.

Then after this, I would put to this Salt by little and little his Mercuriall liquor, which I would diſtill from it, that I might conioyne with the fixed ſalte, the volatile armoniac, which is included in that liquor, and from whome the liquor borroweth his whole force, which I perceyued to be deteyned and ſwallowed vp by the fixed ſalte: for ſo nature imbraceth nature, and like reioyceth with the like, as ſalt with ſalte.

Theſe things thus finiſhed, that is, theſe ſaltes being vnited together againe, then would I adde by little and little the ſulphurous eſſence, which I would bring into earth foliate, that is to ſay : the moſt ſimple eſſence, full of all vitall Tinctures and properties.

But wanting leyſure to go forward in this courſe, I haue not as yet attayned the vndoubted experience of this ſo noble a ſecrete : whereof I will make proofe and aſſaye, if God permit,

G   when

when occafion fhalbe giuen. Fo2 feeing it is a matter in nature, and hath bene alreadie done, there is no doubt but that it may be done againe, by other diligent wo2kemen. Neyther do: I thinke that there can be a mo2e ready way of wo2king p2epa- red, than that which I haue already fpoken of, and which is kno- wen and familiar to true Philofophers, and Chymifts. Fo2 this conrfe obferued, euery thing wel w2ought, hath his moft effectual and actiue uertues, and vital qualities. But fome other better learned and mo2e exercifed in Chymical philofophy then my felfe, can mo2e readily fee this thing, and looke further into the wo2ke- manfhip, who hauing better leyfure, may make trial of this wo2- king, and finde out in very deede the truth and certainty of the ar- tifice. Wherunto if any man by his induftry do attaine, let him not kepe the fecrete to himfelfe alone, but let him beftow the fame vppon men of good parts, fo2 the which benefite they fhal ftand bounde fo2 euer.

Fo2 albeit, it is a matter mo2e pleafant to beholde then p2ofi- table, yet it openeth and awaketh the d2owfie eyes of the mo2e witty and learned fo2t of men, to beholde and take in hande fo2 greatter and mo2e p2ofitable things fo2 mankinde : who after- warde wil guide into the right way, the blinde, and fuch as doe erre th2ough igno2ance, and wil ftoppe the mouthes of euil ton- gued and malicious men.

CHAP. XI.

Concerning the vifible bodies of
the Elements.

IT now refteth that fomewhat bee faide, concerning the vifible Bodies of the Ele- ments, which of all things, as wel of Mine- ral, as of Uegetable, and Animal, doe al- wayes appeare to be two : the one d2ye, the other moyft. The d2ye is a Sandy earth o2 afhes, denoyde of all falt, by reafon of the
washing

washing of Waters, and is called by the *Chymists, Terra dam-*
nata, or Damned earth. Becaufe it hath no other force, but that
which is drying.

The moyfte which is called unfauorie Phleame, is peftered
with all Sulphur and Mercurie, hauing no odour or tafte, or
other vital vertue, which can onely moyften, without any other
force at all.

And as thefe are of no force, fo doe they onely poffeffe
paffiue qualities, and unprofitable. But Ayer, the thyrd Element, cannot be feparated by it felfe, but doth eyther banifh into
ayre, or elfe remayneth mixed Sulphur and Mercury, and doth
more chiefely cleaue unto Mercury, which is fo fpiritual, that the
moft expecte workeman cannot feparate the fame from it felfe
alone, but doth alwayes paffe away into aire, with the aire or
vapour of that thing, whereof the feparation is made : to which
aier Mercury is ftraitely combyned, that it can neuer be feparated from the fame, without it be done by the great induftry of a
fkilful workeman, who knoweth that Mercury or falte Armoniack volatile, is fo conioyned with aier, or with the aiery parte,
that it doth alfo breathe away with the aiery parte, and with the
fame is reduced into fpiritual Water, which is knowen to be the
mercurial water, by the fharpe, fower, and vehement, which
fpringeth from the Mercury or falt armeniack, of nature fpirituall. The which the workeman feeking to feparate, conioy-
neth this fpiritual liquor, with a Chriftalline falt, naturally fixed,
from the which, he feparateth that aiery liquor, by Diftillation,
which by that feparation is utterly fpoyled of all force, and remaineth an unfauory aiery liquor, for becaufe that Mercuriall
fpirite poffeffing the nature of volatil Salt, remaineth fixed,
with his proper Salt, with the which hee hath the moft chiefe
analogie and proportion. And thus the Philofophers teftify,
that nature is delighted with nature.

Thus we fée how the Elementary aier is to be feparated
from that Mercuriall fpirite, namely by bringing the Element
of aier, into water deuoyde of tafte, and by entring the Mercu-

riall

riall fpirit, into the falt, of his proper preheminence.

Furthermore, hereby it appeareth, that Mercury is a certaine airy thing, or aier it felfe: and yet fomewhat more then the elementarie aier, which wanting the fpirit of Mercurie, is a fimple airy liquor of no vertue or power, but fimplie to moyften and penetrate. And fo the actiue qualities doe belong to the beginnings, Salt, fulphur, and Mercurie, and the paffiue to the Elements. This thing wæ haue made plaine before, by the example of Wine, and Water of life. Thefe things are therefore fpoken, that all men may fæ by the Anatomie and refolution of things, that the element of aier, cannot be feparated by it felfe alone, neyther is it fo to be fæne of any, but of the true Philofophers, and by fuch as are moft conuerfant in this art.

Thus certaine demonftration is made of the vifible bodies of things procreated, both out of the fædes and beginnings, and alfo out of the elements; albeit in the refolution of the bodies, thou doeft not difcerne the vifible bodies of the fædes, put a parte by themfelues. But it is an cafie matter to difcerne the feuered partes of thofe thre beginnings, and alfo of the Elements, in the which partes of the thre beginnings, the vertues and powers of actions (wherwith the fædes are moued) are included and mixed together. Whereby it commeth to paffe, that their bodies are filled together with the vitall forces and faculties of the Aftrall and fpirituall fædes, as the receptacle of thofe vertues.

But the Elementall bodies, haue only paffiue qualities: the which elementall bodies, a workeman cannot onely feparate by themfelues, but can alfo bring them to nothing, in fuch forte that the paffiue and materiall Elements being feparated, there fhall onely remaine thofe thre Hypoftaticall, Formall, and Actiue beginnings, falt, fulphur, and mercury, which being drawen into one body, do make a mixed body, which the Philofophers call a fifth or a fourth Effence, which is free from all corruption, abounding with quickening fpirits: whereas contrariwife, the fole elements feparated from thofe thre beginnings, doe bring nothing but impurities, corruptions, and mortification.

In this Chymeftry is to be extolled, that imitating nature, it
fepa

rateth Elements, and their beginnings, by which all the partes of a compound body, are anatomized and made manifest. And yet thofe naturall fubftances, are not faid to be begotten, by fuch feparations, as if they were not before: neyther yet as being before, are they corrupted by the arte of feparation, but they were in compounde, and after feparation, they ceafed not to bee, and to fubfift. And as the three beginnings are coupled together, by the benefite of an oylelie liquor ioyning them in one: fo the three Elements, Ayer, Water, and Earth, are combyned together, by the comming in of Water as a meane. For water by her ana logie and conuenience partaketh both of the nature of aier, and of earth: whereby it commeth to paffe, that one while it is ea fily turned into aier, another while into earth: and fo it comby neth both the extreames. In things that haue likeneffe, an alte ration is eafily made. For, by reafon of likeneffe and confent, aier made thicke with colde, paffeth into water, and water made thinne, becommeth aier: and water alfo made groffe and thick, becommeth earth: euen as earth alfo made thinne, paffeth into water, and is chaunged.

Wherefore, forfomuch as aier and earth, two extreames, are fitlie ioyned together, by a thyrd, which is water, a meane be twæne them both: Ariftotle did more than was næcdefull to ap poynt a quaternarie number of Elements, out of the quaternary number of the fower qualities. Hote, Colde, Drie, Moyft. How beit, it cannot be denied, but that he had great probability hereof, as is to be feene in his fecond booke of the generation of liuing creatures, where he goeth about by many reafons to prœue, that it is moft neceffary for the production of things, to appoynt a fourth element, namely Fyer, hote and drie.

But forfomuch as Mofes in the firft Chapt. of his *Genefis* (wherein he fheweth the creation of all things) maketh no men tion of Fier: it is more conuenient that we leaue it rather to the opinion of the diuine Prophet, then to the reafons of an *Eth nick* Philofopher. And therfore wæ acknowledge no other Fier then Heauen, & the fiery Region which is fo called of burning.

Therefore it ought to be called the fourth formall Heauen,

ant

and essential element, or rather the fourth essence, extracted out of the other elements: bicause it is indued with far more noble vertues, then the most simple elements. For the *Hermeticall Philosophers* deny that there is a quintessence, because there are not fower elements, from whence there may be drawen a fifth essence, but three onely and no more, out of which a fourth may be extracted. So great is the power of this fourth essence, that it moveth, sharpeneth, and mightily animateth the bodies of the three principles, and of the more grosse elements, to come into a perfect mixture of one thing which neuer after can be diuided. Whereupon the Indiuiduals, or simples which cannot be diuided, doe borrow from *Heauen*, & from no other. all those forces, faculties, and properties, which they haue and shewe forth. Hereupon it commeth that the proper qualitie of that essence, is neither drye nor moiste, nor colde, nor hote. For it is a far more simple thing, that is to say, a most simple and pure essence, extracted out of the more simple and more subtil beginnings and elements, which maketh a most simple, most pure, most thinne, and most swifte body, indued with the greatest force of generating, nourishing, increasing, and perfecting, which commeth so neere vnto the nature of fier, that in very deede the *Heauen* is no other thing, but a pure and ethereal fier, neither is the pure fire, any thing els but *Heauen* : which the more it ouercometh the principles and elements, the more it obtaineth, the more potent, perfect, pure, and simple forces and vertues, by which it pearceth into all things, and furnisheth euery thing with his formes and vertues.

It appeareth therefore by *Moses*, that there is no other fiery Element, but *Heauen*, which hath the place of the fourth element, or which is rather a fourth essence extracted out of the more subtil matter and forme of the three elements, which is no other thing, but a pure ethereal, and most simple fier, most perfect, and most far different, from the three elements, as imperfite: which fier, is the author of all formes powers, and actions in all the inferior things of nature, as the first cause, and carrying it selfe like the parent, toward his offspring: which fier, by his winde carryeth & conueyeth his seedes into the belly of the earth, whereby the gene-

ration

The Heauen of Philoso-phers.

ration o₂ fruite is nouriſhed, foſtered, groweth and is at the laſt thruſt to₂th, out of the lappe o₂ boſome of the elements.

This *Heauen*, albeit in it ſelfe, it is no complexion, that is to ſay, neither hote no₂ cold, no₂ moyſt, no₂ d₂ie : yet by his knowledge and p₂edeſtination, it yældeth to all things, heate and colde, moyſtneſſe, and d₂yneſſe : fo₂ſomuch as there are ſtarres which haue their moſt colde and moyſt ſpirites, as the *Saturnalls* , and *Lunaries* : others, moſt hote and d₂ie, as the *Solarie*, and *Martialls* : others hote and meyſt, as the *Iouialls,* who by their vertues and complexion (wherwith euery Starre and Planet is inbued) do info₂me, faſhion, ⁊ imp₂egnat all theſe inferio₂ things, in ſuche wiſe, that ſome indiuidualls are of this condicion and complexion, which they haue bo₂rowed and taken from their info₂ming o₂ faſhioning planet o₂ ſtarre : other ſome of that which they haue obtained from other Planets and Starres. Fo₂ God hath giuen to *Heauen* moſt ſimple and perfect ſæces, ſuch as are the Starres and Planets, which hauing in them Vitall faculties, and complexions, do powze them fo₂th into the lappe of the inferio₂ Elements and do animate and fo₂me them. Neyther doth the *Heauen* ceaſſe from his wo₂king, no₂ the *Aſtrall* ſæces therof, becauſe their vertues are neuer exhauſted : neyther do they ſuffer alteration o₂ diminution of faculties, wherby they may ceaſſe from procreating o₂ fo₂ming, albeit that ſometime they do make mo₂e o₂ leſſe fruitfull then at other ſome. Herevpon commeth that perpetuall Circulation, by the benefite whereof the ſæces of the Elements o₂ they₂ matter, are coupled with the ſæedes of the Starres, ſetting and putting their contayned into the maternall lappe, that it may fo₂me and b₂ing fo₂th a kindly ſp₂out. Fo₂ as *Heauen* is ſayde to wo₂ke vppon the *Earth* , ſo alſo the inferio₂ Elements , do yælde and beſtowe their actions and motions, but not after one manner : fo₂ that *Heauen* in acting ſuffereth nothing, ſo farre fo₂th as it is equalled, being of a Homogeniall and moſt perfect nature : and therefo₂e is inco₂ruptible and Immutable vnto the p₂edeſtinated ende of things created.

But theſe inferio₂ things do ſuffer in their action , becauſe they haue they₂ fo₂mall beginnings , mixed with their materialls,

rialls, subiect to chaunge and destruction: whereuppon also it commeth to passe, that those things which proceede from them, do in continuance of time decay and perish.

These things knowen to a true Phisitian and Philosopher, hée séeketh to restore decayed health, and to preserue the same by the extraction of celestiall Essences and Formes, and the elementarie separation of the beginnings and materialls, from those thrée formall and spirituall beginnings, the which he vseth alone, separated from the others, which are Heterogeniall, or of another kinde, that he may worke wonderful effects without any impediment.

And this is the vniuersal Ballamick medecine, wherin all the partes are Homogeneal, or of one kinde most pure, most simple, and most spirituall, And being in such simplicitie, and most thoroughly clensed and purged from all grosse Feces, and incorrupt, it is called a Quintessence, but more truly and properly a Quartessence, and the celestial stone of the Philosophers.

But let no man thinke here, that when I name the Philosophers stone, (that is to say, that vniuersal medicine) that I meane the transmutation of metalls, as if such transmutation, were the chéefe medicine of mans body: but knowe rather, that in Man, (which is a little world) there lye hidde the mynes of Imperfect metals, from whence so many diseases do growe, which by a good faithful and skilful Phisittian must be brought to Golde and Siluer, that is to say, vnto perfect purification, by the vertue of so excellent a medicine, if we wil haue good and prosperous health.

The Phisittian therefore, must diligently consider two things, that is to saye, that Nature may be disquieted, both by an inward and also by an outward enemie. But this more especially he must foresée, that Nature be not tormented with the outward enemie. which then commeth to passe, when a medecine is ministred and giuen, which is crude, impure, and venimous, and therefore contrary to our nature and spirites. Then on the other side, he must haue care that the domesticall enemies which are within mans body, be dryuen out with conuenient and fitte weapons. For if a remedy be applyed which is vnfitte, then Nature is aſſayled by two enemies, that is to ſay, by the externall medicine, and by the inwarde impuritie, which remaining long in the body, turneth into poyſon, if ſpeedy remedy be not had.

CHAP. XII.

Moſes in his Geneſis ſheweth the three beginnings Philoſophicall which are in euery thing created.

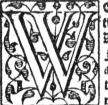 E holde by *Moſes* doctrine, that *G O D* in the beginning made of nothing a *Chaos*, or Deepe, or Waters, if wee pleaſe ſo to call it. From the which Chaos, Deepe, or waters, animated with the Spirite of God, God as the great workemaiſter and Creator, ſeparated firſt of all *Light* from *Darkeneſſe*. and this *Æthereall Heauen*, which wee beholde, as a fifth Eſſence, or moſt pure Spirite, or moſt ſimple ſpirituall body. Then hee diuided Waters, from Waters; that is to ſay, the more ſubtill, Aiery, and *Mercuriall* liquor, from the more Thicke, Clammy, and Oylely, or Sulphurous liquor. After that, he extracted and brought foorth the *Sulphur*, that to ſay, the more groſſe Waters, from the drye parte, which out of the ſeparation ſtandeth like ſalte, and as yet ſtandeth by it ſelfe apart. And yet for all this, thoſe vniuerſall partes of the whole *Chaos*, are not to be ſeparated, but that ſtil euery one of them, do retaine in themſelues, thoſe three beginnings without the which they cannot bee, nor yet fulfill their generations. This was the worke of God, that hee might ſeparate the Pure from the Impure: that is to ſay, that he might reduce the more pure and Æthereal Mercury, the more pure and inextinguible Sulphur, the more pure, and more fired ſalte, into ſhyning and inextinguible Starres and Lights, into a Chriſtalline and Dyamantine ſubſtance, or moſt ſimple Bodie, which is called *Heauen*, the higheſt, and fourth formall Element, and that from the ſame, the Formes as it were ſeedes, might be

D   pow

powred forth into the most grosse elements, to the generation of all things. The which are called the more grosse elements, because from them in the diuision of the *Chaos*, the most pure part is abstracted and conuerted and brought to a heauen, and to the fruites thereof.

All which elements whether it be that most simple fourth, or whether they be those, which are said to be more grosse, forso, much as they consist of those three Hypostaticall beginning, they could neuer be so separated one from the other at the first, nor can now bee so seperated by any *Chymist*, but that alwayes still that which remaineth is compounded of them three. The difference is this, that some are most pure, simple, and most spirituall substances of the secret parts, and other some are more grosse and lesse simple, also a third sort, most grosse and material in the highest degree.

Therefore it must be confessed, that the Heauen, albeit it bee most simple, doth consist of those three beginnings, but of the most pure and most spirituous, and altogether formall. Whereby it commeth to passe, that the vertues and powers of Heauen, being wholy spirituall, doe easily without impediment pearcing into the other Elements, powre forth the interiour Elements the spirituall formes: from whence all mortall bodies doe obtaine the increase both of their vertues, and also of their faculties.

If we will behold the puritie of the Heauen aboue other Elements, and the perpetuall constancie thereof, looke then vpon those bright and shining tyers, continually glittering and light, to whom the heauen hath giuen the most pure and extinguible substance of Sulphur, whereof they consist. For such as the heauen is in essence, such and the like fruites hath it brought foorth in substance: out of whose vitall impressions and influences, they procreat bring foorth some likenes of theselues, in the more grosse Elemets: but yet accoding as the matter is more grosse or more thinne, more durable or more constant, or more transitorie.

And the influences of such tyers, are mercuriall spirits: but the light and shyning brightnes, is Sulphur: their fixed Heauens, or Aitriall and Chrystallyne circles, is a salt body: which
circles,

circles, are so pure, shining and fixed, that a Diamond which partaketh of the nature of fixed salt, is not of moze puritie, continuance and perpetuitie than they are.

As touching the Elements of Ayer, the beginnings thereof are moze grosse, lesse pure, and lesse spirituall and simple, than the beginnings celestiall, and yet much moze perfect, thinne, and penetrating, then are the waterie and terrestriall Mercuries and Sulphurs: and is such, that next to heauen it hath the preheminence of actiuitie and power, whose forces are to be seene in diuers and sundzy windes which are mercuriall fruites and the spirits of the ayerie Element: whose sulphurs also are discerned to be pure and bzight in burning Comets, which are no perpetuall fires oz sulphurs, which cannot bee put out loz degenerating from the nature of Celestiall starres and Sulphurs, as from puritie & simplicitie, into a moze grosse and impure fozme.

Now as concernining Earth which is ayerie, it is so subtill and thinne, that it is very hard to be seene, being diffused thzoughout the whole Region of the Ayer: which doth not sent it selfe to the eye, but in Mannas, in Delwes, and in Frostes, as in aierie salts. The verie same beginnings of ayer, may also be seene in Meteozs: which in it, and out of it, are ingendered, that is to say, in lightnings, in cozruscations, and in thunderings, & in such like. Foz in that fierie flame which bzeaketh fozth is Sulphur: In the windy spirit, & moystnesse is Mercury: au in the thunderbolt oz stone of the lightning, is salt fixed.

The fruites also of this nature are Manna celestiall, and hony, which Bees do gather from flowers, wherein there is no other thing but Salt, Sulphur, and Mercurie of the ayer: which by a skilfull wozkeman are not separated from those without great admiration: yea the rustick *Coridon* findeth this by experience to be true, when as he can seperate the matter of the Bees wozke, into waxe, which is a matter sulphurus, into hony, which is a Mercurial essence, & into dzosse, repzesenting the terrestriall salte. And thus that superioz globe seuered into an ethereall and ayery heauen, hath his thzee beginnings, yet neuerthelesse very different in simplicitie and puritie.

E 2   CAHP.

CHAP. XIII.

Whence is fhewed, that in this inferior Globe of the Worlde, namely in the Elements of Water and Earth, thefe three beginnings are plainely to be feene.

Hofe th2ee Beginnings, doe as yet mo2e plainely fhewe-fo2th themfelues in this inferio2 Globe, by reafon of their mo2e groffe matter, which is to our eyes mo2e fenfible. Fo2 out of the Element of Water, the iuy-ces and metallick fubftances do daily b2eak fo2th in fight: the vapours of whofe moyfture o2 iuyce mo2e fpirituous, do fet fo2th *Mercury*: the mo2e d2ye exhalations, *Sulphur*: and their roagulated o2 congealed matter, Salt. Of the which faltes Nature doth offer vnto vs dyuers kindes of Allume, of Vitriole, (fund2y differences, Salte-gemme, and falt Armoniac, and many others. Th2re are alfo manie kindes of Sulphurs, of Pitche, and of Bitumen, and of Mercuries, o2 Juyces. Mo2eouer the Sea doth witnes, that it is not without fuch Mercuriall, Aiery and Sulphurous fpirites: whofe meteo2s in *Caftor* and *Pollux*, and in other ftars kindled, by reafon of their fund2y fulphurs and exhalations, do confirme the fame: and that the fea is not without his faltes, the faltneffe thereof doth make manifeft. The Earth, alfo doth p2oue the fame, which being like vnto a fpunge, doth continually d2aw and fucke vnto it the falte body thereof: Wherby it cometh to paffe, that there are fo many kindes of metalls and Mineralls therin. From this Marine falte, as from the Father and firft o2iginal, all other fates are deryued. And thefe beginnings are fo fepara-ted in all other Elementes by themfelues aparte, that no one of them is dep2yued of the company of another. Fo2 in the Marine falte, albeit the nature of falte, doth exc�de and ouermatche the nature of the other beginnings, yet it is not deftitute of a fulphurous and mercuriall effence, as by *Chymicall* experience may be.

Chymicall Phyſicke.

be made plaine. Fo2 he which is a meane *Chymiſt* knoweth how to extracte out of the ſame by the fo2ce of fire, a ſharpe Mercuriall ſpirite, which being Ethereall, and therefo2e moſte Potente, doth diſſolue into liquo2, the moſt firme and harde metall, as Galde, which otherwiſe cannot be ouercome neither with the moſt vehement fyer, no2 bæ conſumed with any long continuance of time.

Furthermo2e, a wo2keman knoweth how to extract out of the ſame ſalt, congealed ſtones, very ſweete, and of a Sulphurus nature, which neuertheleſſe haue a mightie and admirable fo2ce, to diſſolue the moſt hard thing that is. And yet fo2 all this, that which remaineth is Salt. Thus you ſee plainely that theſe th2æ beginings, Salt, Sulphur, and Mercury, are contained in the Marine Salt.

The ſame alſo is to be ſæne Uitriol, the which among other Salts is moſt co2po2eat. Fo2 alwayes fo2 the moſt part figures and Images of *Venus* and *Mars*, are to be ſæne therein and conioyned together.

Venus and Mars are Copper and Iron.

In this Uitriol, I ſay, doe plainely appeare, Salt, Sulphur, and Mercurie. Whoſe Mercurie altogether ethereall, being by art ſeparated, and made moſt pure, from the elementary paſſiue flegme, poſſeſſeth a græne ſharpe ſpirit, of ſo great an acting and penetrating fo2ce, that in a very ſho2t time it will diſſolue metalyne bodyes, and moſt hard ſubſtances, whether they be mettals o2 ſtones. And this is that græne Lyon, which *Rypley* commendeth ſo much.

The greene von.

The Sulphur in Uitriol, is eaſily diſcerned by a certaine red Dcre, ſweet, which is eaſily ſeparated from the ſame: which is an aſſwager of things, and a right actatiue, and a great mittigato2 all griefes, and paines.

But the Colcotar, o2 red feces with remayneth in the bottome, after the ſeperation of the ethereall Mercury, and of the ſwæte Sulphur, conteyned in it, a moſt white Salt, the extraction whereof maketh a very good and gentle vomit, fit and p2ofitable fo2 many diſeaſes.

As theſe th2æ are found in Uitriol, ſo alſo they are to be found

in

in Allum,and in other Salts,as we haue shewed before concerning common Salt.

    They are also to be seene in common Sulphur, wherein be-
side the Sulphurus substance, and inflamable matter, there is
contained a Mercuriall sharpish liquor, so pearcing, that it is a-
ble to open and vnlock the most strong and hard gates of *Sol*
and L*una*.

    But the Salt drawen from the other parts, remaineth in the
bottome,as euery meane workman knoweth. And such is this
sowerish spirit of Sulphur,that although it be drawen out of Sulphur, fit to burne,yet it is so vnfit to take fier, that it is easily let
from burning.

    It happeneth otherwise to common Mercurie , which is al-
together ethereall and spirituall : (from whence the third beginning of all things which is most spirituall , hath borrowed the
name, albeit it is not like vnto common Mercurie, or to quick-
siluer in forme), For out of the same, both a liquor,and a sweete
Sulphur,and also a Salt may be extracted.

    Hereby it is easily iudged, that these three principles of Chy-
mists are not the common Salt, Sulphur, and Mercurie : but
some other thing of nature,more pure and simble, which neuerthelesse hath some conscience and agreement with common Salt,
Sulphur,and Mercurie: from whence also our beginnings haue
taken their name: and not without cause , for that the common
are in all mixt things, and in all things most simple and spirituall. For the other being mixed with the more grosse substances
of bodies,are hindered from being so volatile and spirituall. For
that they consist of many vnkindly parts , with the which these
common spirits are not so holden backe.

    Of those three beginnings aforesaid, all metalls are compoun-
ded,albeit after diuers sorts. And this is the cause,that they differ so much one from an other. For in pron, the Sulphur thereof
which may be burnt, in that it passeth almost away in sparkes &
sinders by meanes of the fier, doth exceed in qualitie the other
two beginnings, and doth ouersway them : Hereof it commeth,
that will be on fier throughout . For the which cause it is called
by

by the old Philoſophers,by the name of the Planet *Mars*,a bur∕
ning Planet.

So copper hath great ſtoze of Sulphur,but leſſe burning then
that of pzon,and it hath alſo much vitriol ſalt,yet but little quan∕
titie of Mercurie.But that vitriolated Salt, is that ſharpe fer∕
ment of nature, whereby the generations of all naturall things
are propagated and increaſed: whereupon the name of *Venus* is
giuen to Copper:in whom there is a ſecond quaternarie among
the Planets, where are heaped vp, nouriſhed, and coagulated
ſpiritually all celeſtiall eſſences:wherefoze this Planet by all the
auncient Philoſophers is called *Venus*, the mother of generati∕
ons, and begotten of the males froth.

Tiane hath in it much ethereall and aiery Mercury, but of
combuſtible Sulphur,a ſmall quantitie, and the leaſt poztion of
Salt.And hereof it commeth that Philoſophers call the ſame *Iu∕
piter*,becauſe that Planet is altogether aiery and ethereall : and
therefoze Poets appoint him king of the aier, and the region of
lightning.

Gold and ſiluer,which of all other metalls are moſt noble and
perfit,do alſo conſiſt of the thzee fozeſaid beginnings,but yet mix∕
ed in equalitie, and ſo perfetly with great purity vnited,that it
may ſeeme that there is one chiefe and firſt eſſence onely in them,
and not thzee,of which they conſiſt. Foz theyz *Salt*, *Sulphur*,and
Mercury, are ſo ſtraitly ,and by the leaſt things ſo ioyned toge∕
ther, that it may ſeeme they are one ſubſtance, not thzee,oz con∕
ſiſting of thzee.

Notwithſtanding moſt pure *Mercury* , ſeemeth to excell and
ouerſway in ſiluer, by which it is made moze moyſt then Golde,
which is the moſt temperate of all other.

But in Golde, the ſulphur which is fired and incombuſtible,
of a fiery nature, bzingeth to paſſe that it ſtandeth inuincible a∕
gainſt all fozce of fier , and loſeth not the leaſt waite thereof,be∕
cauſe like wil neuer oppzeſſe his like,but contrariwiſe do cheriſh
and pzeſerue one the other : whereby it commeth to paſſe
that it ioyeth in the fier , and alwaies commeth out of
the ſame, moze pure and noble then it went in . Therefoze
the.

the name of the Sunne is giuen to gold, becaufe in very dæde it is an ethereall fier and b2ightneffe. Fo2 the Sunne is a moft fiery fhining Planet, giuing to all things, by his heat and fpirits, life. But filuer fo2 the fo2ce and p2opertie of Mercuriall humiditie which it hath with the Moone, a Planet full of radicall moyfture and p2egnant, is called by the name of the Moone.

Leade containeth much Salt, and great plentie of indigefted and crude Mercury, but leffe flying Sulphur : hereupon it commeth, that lead is the examiner of all other metalls, which it difperceth into fume, as is to be féene by tryall , excepting the two perfect metalls, gold and filuer, which it cannot confume.

This vertue of confuming the bodies of imperfect metalls it hath from that qualitie of Crude and flying Mercury , with the which it doth abound : whereas otherwife by the nature of his Sulphur, it is able to doe the contrarie: that is to fay, to coagulate thofe metallick fpirits, and to reduce them into bodies, euen as quickfiluer being altogether flying by nature, etheriall, and truly Homogeny and fpirituall, both after a fo2t congeale and fire. So that hereby it appeareth, that it hath in it by nature, the fpirit of heat and of cold, and therefo2e of metallick life and death : which maketh the fentence of *Hermes* good, when he faid, that which is aboue, is all one with that which is beneath. Fo2 fuch as is Saturne in the fuperio2 Elements, fuch alfo is lead in the inferiour: and fo of the reft.

And out of that burning licquo2, mo2e ready to burne, then the very Aquauitie, may be feperated a Mercurie, o2 a mo2e ethereall fpirit by a Matraf with a long necke, by a gentle fier. The which fo feperated , the reft of the matter of meane fubftance, which is Sulphurus, Oylely, and apt to burne, refteth in the bottome of the glaffe , with the Niterous and Sulphurus fpirit of Salt.

Out of the blacke feces, which remaine in the bottome of the reto2t, being reduced acco2ding to the Phylofophicall maner into a calye, is extracted a fixed Salt , which often times diffolued and Coagulated with his p2oper fleame , will at the laft become Ch2yftalline.

To this, if there be afterward powred by little and little according to Art, his ethereal ſpirit, that from hence it may contract and drawe the double or triple waight of the volatile, and truly Mercurial ſalt, in ſuch wiſe that being caſt vpon a red hote plate, it doe diſpearce into fume: thou ſhalt at the laſt, by the means of ſublimation, attaine to the foliat earth of the Phyloſophers, which will haue a greater brightneſſe and perſpicuitie, then can be ſeene in the moſt rich and orient pearle in the world. This earth the Phyloſophers call their Mercurie the which alone hath admirable properties and faculties.

Againe, if to this be added the oylely liquor of his proper Sulphur alſo exalted and kept a part by it ſelfe, in a iuſt & conuenient qualitie, and if the ſame be drawen forth with ſundry cohobations and extillations, againe and againe, repeated and iterated, and be reaffunded and diſtilled, vntil out of a Ternarie, there ariſe a vnitie: then out of the groſſe, terreſtrial: and material lead, ſhal ariſe and ſpring vp a certaine celeſtial and true diſſoluer of nature, and a quinteſſence of admirable vertue and efficacie: the true, liuely, and cleare ſhyning fountaine wherein (as Poets affirme, hyding vnder a vaile their ſecrets) *Vulcan* waſhed *Phebus*, and which clenſeth away all impuritie, to make a moſt pure and perfect body, repleniſhed with vital ſpirits, and full of vegetation: and doth ſo rid himſelfe from his adamantine fetters with the which he was bound, and hindered from the victorie againſt the Serpent *Pytho*, and doth in ſuch wiſe ſhake off all impediments, that being free from all duſkie cloudes of darkeneſſe, with the which he was couered and ouerwhelmed, he ſendeth forth now vnto vs his moſt bright ſhining light, with the which wee are throughly refreſhed, receyuing youthful ſtrength, putting off all imbecillitie, and like vnto that *Aſon* king of *Creta*, through the helpe of *Media*, are throughly reſtored againe to young age. So that the ſame thing which afore was altogether cold without blood, and denoided of life ſeeming as dead, being waſhed in this fountaine, it ariſeth and triumpheth in glory, in might, and furniſhed with all vertues, and accompanied with an exceeding army of ſpirits, doth communicate vnto vs freely his glory and

J
brightneſſe,

brightneſſe, and doth moſt mightily reſtoze and cozrobozate the
ſtrength of our radicall balſome, with his onely looke and touch,
thzoughly weeding and rooting out all the cauſes and ſeedes of
ſickneſſes lurking in vs, and ſo conſuming them, that without al
trouble, it pzeſerueth our helth, vnto the appointed end of our life.

He which hath eares to heare let him heare attentiuely, otherwiſe let him neuer take his wozke in hand. Foz albeit I haue
ſhewed the way to perfect wozking moze plainely (as I thinke)
then any other hitherto haue done, yet thou mayeſt erre except
thou be wholely addicted and intent to thy wozke.

Thus the way is pzepared foz true Phyloſophers, to attaine
to that great and moſt excellent minerall wozke, and to the pzeparing of that vniuerſal medicine out of mineralls. And this is
the demonſtration, by which in all metalls and concrete bodies,
thoſe thzee beginnings are to be ſearched out, and being by art
ſeperated, are to be ſet befoze our eyes. The which to make it
moze plaine, I thought good to vſe the example of lead, which of
all men is reiected as moſt vile, whereas notwithſtanding the
Phyloſophers haue the ſame in great eſteeme, becauſe they ful
wel know, what great ſecrets it containeth within. And therefoze they cal it their Sunne oz leperous gold.

From this tree of _Saturne_ ſpzingeth Antimony, as the firſt
bzanch of the ſtock, which the Phyloſophers cal their Magneſia,
which aboue all other metallick ſubſtances, containeth theſe thzee
beginnings ful of open actiuitie and efficacie. _Paracelſus_ among
all other Chymical Phyloſophers, hath wonderfully ranſacked
all the parts thereof, and examined the beginnings moſt diligently, whoſe ſubſtance he hath exalted and commended, aboue
al other metallick ſubſtances, and eſpecially the Mercury therof:
out of which, as out of the chiefeſt ſubiect, and moze noble matter, he wzought his chiefeſt and beſt wozks. In the pzaiſe wherof, theſe are _Paracelſus_ own wozds: Antimony is the true balme
of gold, which the Phyloſophers cal the examiner. And the Poets faine that _Vulcan_ waſhed _Phœbus_ in the ſame lauer, and purged him from al his ſpots and imperfections, being deriued from
moſt pure and perfect Mercury and Sulphur, vnder a kinde of
Vitriol,

Uitriol,into a metallick forme and brightneſſe. Hee compareth the ſame alſo in an other place to the matter of gold,concerning whoſe vertues and effects he deliuereth wonders : as that it is the higheſt and moſt perfect purger of gold,and his Mercury,of men.His red Sulphur alſo doth plainly appeare,which hath his property,that it wil take fier and burne like common Sulphur or Brimſtone:the which is eſpecially to be ſene in the night,ꝗ in a darke place,without any fume, which the common Sulphur is woont to ſend forth. This Sulphur of Antimony is Solary,and ſuch as is able to gild the ſuperficial part of ſiluer.

As touching the Salt of Antimony, it is to be ſeperated from the ſame,whoſe property conſiſteth in procuring vomit.For his ſtrength to procure vomit lyeth hid in the ſalte flowers thereof: from the which flowers, if the ſalt betaken away ꝗ ſeperated by vertue of a certaine ſalt,as may be done,then out of the flowers thereof,is made a moſt excellent purgation without vomiting.

But the property of the Mercury thereof bringeth no ſmal wonder , which in the liquation or melting of gold with other metalls,reiecteth them al , and chooſeth the gold to it ſelfe, with the which it is mingled and vnited into one body , in ſuch wiſe, that it ſwalloweth vp gold,whereas all other metalls (except ſiluer)do floate aloft, and wil not ſinke into the ſame . Conſider therefore , (ſaith *Arnold*,) that thing onely which cleaueth to Mercury and to the perfect bodies , and thou haſt the full knowledge.And when he hath thus diſcribed the deuouring Ly-on,he addeth theſe words: Becauſe our ſtone is like to the occidentall quickſiluer, which carrieth gold before it,and ouercommeth it:and is the very ſame which can kill and make aliue.And know further,that our coagulated quickſiluer,is the father of all the minerals of that our magiſtery,ꝗ is both body ꝗ ſpirit, *&c.*

The ſame three chiefe beginnings , doe offer themſelues vnto vs in other ſemi mineralls, as in Arſenick, orpiment,and ſuch other like: which albeit in their whole ſubſtance they bee contrary to our nature and ſpirits , yet by nature they haue that ſpiritual promptnes , and flying ſwiftneſſe, that by their ſubtiltie , they eaſily conuey and mingle

I 2   [them-

and mingle themfelues with our fpirits , whether they be inwardly taken,oz outwardly applyed, and doe wozke venemous
and moztal effects,and that by reafon of the Arfenical Mercury
poinfon ful,oz arfenical Sulphur,and arfenicall Salt.

Gems alfo and pzecious ftones , haue in them the vertues
and qualities of thofe thzee beginnings : by reafon of whofe fier
ant bzightnefle, the pure Mercury in them doth fhine, cleaning
firmly to his fixed Salt, and alfo to the Sulphur of the fame nature , whereby the whole fubftance of a contrary kind being feperated , there arifeth and is made a moft pure ftone of contri-
uance like vnto gold.

Of this fozt is the moft firme and conftant Diamond , to
whom that good old Saturne hath giuen the leaden colour of his
moze pure Mercury, together with the fixed and conftant fpirits of his moze pure Sulphur, and hath fo confirmed, conica-
led and compacted it in all ftability,with his chziftalline falt, that
of all other ftones it is the moft folyd and hardeft , by reafon of
the moft firme vnion of the thzee pzincipal beginnings and their
coherence : which by no art of feparation can be diffoyned and
fundered into the folution of his fpiritual beginnings.And this is
the caufe, that the ancient Phyfitians had no vfe thereof in medicine, becaufe it could not be diffolued into his firft matter.

And it is not to be thought , that thofe auncient Phyfitians
reftrained the vfe thereof, foz that they deemed it to be venemous
by nature, (as fome falfely imagin)which being homogenial and
of a moft fimple nature,it is wholely celeftial,and therefoze moft
pure,and foz that caufe nothing venemous: but the poyfon and
daunger commeth here hence,that being onely bzoken and beaten,and in no fozt apt to pzeperation , taken fo into the ftomack,
and remaining there by reafon of his folicitie and hardnefle in-
concocted,by continuance of time,and by little and little, it doth
fret and teare the laps of the ftomack , and fo the intralls being
excoziated,death by a lingering confumption enfueth.

It belongeth to golde, with his Sulphur, to giue a red tincture, to Carbuncles,and Rubines, neither doth the difference of
their colours come of any other caufe, then this, that their
Mercuries

Mercuries and Chryſtallyne ſalts, are not deſeked and clenſed alike: the which clenſing, the more perfect or imperfect it is, the colour appeareth accordingly, either better, or worſe.

And albeit Siluer be outwardly white, yet within, it hath the colour of Azure and blewe, by which ſhee giueth her tincture to Saphyrs.

Copper, hauing outwardly a ſhew of rednes, hath a greene colour within, (as the _Viridgreeſe_ that is made thereof doth teſtiſie,) by which it giueth greenneſſe vnto the _Emeraud._

Iron, red within, as his Saffron & yeallow colour doth plainly ſhew (and yet, nothing like the colour which gold hath within it) giueth colour to the _Iacint._

Tinne, albeit it is earthie, yet being partaker of the celeſtiall nature, it giueth vnto Agates, diuers, and ſundry colours.

From gold, and from other mettals, as alſo from precious ſtones, their colours may be taken away, by Cementation and Reuerberation, by their proper menſtrues, which things are well knowen to _Chymiſts_ and fire workmen. The which colours and ſulphurs ſo extracted, are very fit for the affects of the braine. The colour of gold, ſerueth for the affects of the heart. The colour of tinne, for the lunges. The colour of Mercury, The colour of lead, for the ſplene. The colour of Iron, for the redneſſe. The colour of Copper, for the priuie parts.

The heauenly menſtrueſe, to diſpoyle mettalls of their colours and ſulphures naturall is this: namely the deaw which falleth in the moneth of May, and his ſugar Manna: out of the which two, mixed together, digeſted, and diſtilled according to Arte, there wil come forth a general diſſoluer, moſt fit to diſpoyle ſtones and mettals of their colours. Yea, of onely Sugar, or of hony by it ſelfe, may be made a diſſoluer of mettals.

Now if theſe three beginnings, Salt, Sulphur, and Mercurie, are to be found in the Heauen, in the Ayer, and in the Waters, as is already ſhewed, who wil make any doubt, but that by a farre greater reaſon they are to be found in the earth, and to be made no leſſe apparant, ſeeing the earth of al other elements, is the moſt fruitfull and plentiful.

The Mercurial fpirits fhewe themfelues in the leaues and fruites; The Sulphurus, in the flowers, feedes, and kirnels: The falts, in the wood, barke and rootes: and yet fo, that eache one of thofe thꝛee partes of the trꝍ oꝛ plant, feuerally by them-felues, albeit to one is giuen the mercurial fpirit, to another that of Sulphur, and to the third that of Salt, yet euery one apart, may as yet be refolued into thofe thꝛee beginnings: without the which they cannot confift, how fimple fo euer they be. Foꝛ whatfoeuer it bꝍ, that hath being, within the whole compaſſe and courfe of nature, doe confift, and are pꝛofited by thefe thꝛꝍ beginnings.

And whereas fome are faid to be mercurial, fome Sulphu-rus, and fome Salt, it is therefoꝛe, becaufe the Mercurials doe conteine moꝛe Mercurie, the Sulphurus moꝛe Sulphur, and the Saltiſh moꝛe Salt in them than the others. Foꝛ fome whole trꝍs are to be fꝍne moꝛe fulphurus and rofeny than other fome, as the Pine and Firre-trꝍs, which are alwayes grꝍene in the coldeſt mountaines, becaufe they abound with their Sulphu-rus beginning, being the pꝛincipal vital inſtrumēt of their grow-ing. Foꝛ there are fome other plants, as the Lawꝛel, and the Trꝍs of Oꝛanges, Citrons and Lemons, which continue long grꝍene, and yet are fubiect to colde: becaufe their Sulphure is not fo eafily difperfed, as is the Sulphur of the firre trꝍs, which are rofeny, and are therefoꝛe thꝛice of a moꝛe fixed and conſtant life, furniſhed againſt the iniuries of times. Furthermoꝛe, al Spice trꝍs, and al fragrant and odoꝛiferous hearts are Sulphu-rus. And as there are fundꝛy foꝛtes of trꝍs of this kinde, fo are there an infinite foꝛt of Sulphurs, of the which to entreate here is no place.

There are other Plants which fhew foꝛth Salt: which is to be found and felt by their taſte: as *Celadine, Nettell, Aron,* o-therwife called *Weake Robin, Radiſh, Muſtardſeed, Porret,* oꝛ *Leekes, Garlick, Ramfoms, Perſicaria,* oꝛ *Arfefmart:* which al-fo by the vertue and plenty of their falt, doe defend themfelues from the wrongs of times.

Ros Solis (fo called) aboundeth with Mercurie amongſt other
Mercurial

Mercuriall plants. The which beginning notwithstanding, for so much as it is flging and spirituall, except it be reteined by another moze cozpozeat, that is to say, by a waterie oz aierie liquoz, it vanisheth quite out of sight. But being dismembred & thorough ly searched by the Art of *Chymistrie*, in his interioz Anatomy, with the separation of the beginnings, it may also be made subiect to sense. For Mercury is extracted out of euery thing, first of all in his dissection oz separation, into a watery vapour: and Sulphur into an oyely: thirdly, out of the remaining feces, brought into ashes, a Salt is extracted, by his proper water, which being most white, & like to crystall, hath the taste of sharpe, sower, & byting salt, oz such like relish in the mouth: whereby it is found to be true salte, which may be dissolued in water, accozding to the maner of true salts: differing so much from the other ashes, as life from death: foz as much as the feces that remaine there of, are called dead earth, whereas this is replenished with vitall actions.

To conclude, in euery kind of plant, & in all the partes thereof, thrise three beginnings are inset and cleauing, indued with sundzy properties and faculties, accozding to the varietie of Plants. The which also a skilfull Phisitian vseth diuersly, that he may fit each one to other, accozding to equalitie of matching, and accozding to his intended purpose.

Hereby it appeareth how necessarie the knowledge of the internall Anatomy of things, which shew easily by the impression of things, their properties & vertues, which we may appzoue & confirme by experience. Let vs take foz example, the oyle oz Sulphur of the Boxe-tree, allwayes greene and vitriolated, by whose vnpleasant odour, the stupefactiue Sulphur which is in it, repzesenteth it selfe vnto vs. That oyle, I say, of the Boxe, albeit it wil easily burne, yet is a great asswager and mittigatoz of all paines, as comming nere to the nature and-pzopertie of narcotti call oz stupefactiue sulphur vitriolated, being as auailable against the falling sicknesse as Vitriol.

If we consider the properties of the beginnings of *Camphyre*, it wil manifestly appeare, (although it do burne in water) by his vnpleasaunt odour, that it hath a cooling pzopertie in it, and narco narcocal or ftupefactiue : whofe oyle alfo, is a good mittigator of paines and griefe : when as notwithstanding it sheweth foorth contrary effects, as at the very first brunt, it seemeth to haue a certaine fierie qualitie. By reason of the propertie which it hath to affwage paines and aches, the *Arabians* iudged the fame to colde in the third degrée. The experience thereof is eafily to bée féene in the ache of the téeth. For if a hollow or rotten toothe, bée but touched with the oyle thereof, it putteth away the paine. The fame oyle is a moft prefent remedie in paines and griefe of the reynes, caufed by the ftone. For thereby the ftone is diffolued and auoyded, if it be miniftred with competent liquor.

Other are the properties of other Oyles : For the oyles or Sulphurs of Annis, and of Fennel, are fit to difpearce and driue away windineffe.

The Oyles of Cloues, of Nutmegges, of Cinamon, and of other fpices and their Sulphurs, as alfo the Oyles of Mynts, of *Ambrofia*, of *Sage*, and *Betony*, and of fuch like, are conuenient to corroborat, and to warme the braine and ftomach.

So the ole of Pepper, doth attennat, make thinne, diffolue and cut tartarus matters in the body, and humours that are niter Sulphurus and Cholerick. And howfoeuer many dœe déeme the fame to be hote, yet it is farre more conuenient to bée giuen in cholericke feuers, and to put away other griefes, as tertians, and fuch like, than any other altering or cooling firrupe.

In like fort hote and burning oyles, may be extracted out the féedes of Poppey, Gowrdes, Melons, Cucumbers, and fuch like cold things, whofe operations notwithftanding doe not bring heate, but rather reft and comfortable refrefhing.

And the mercurial fpirits of vegetables, are oftentimes conioyned with fulphurus fpirits : fo that out of *Teribinthine*, which is almoft wholy fulphurus, as alfo out of Pitch and Rofen a mercuriall fpirit, or fharpe liquor, may bée by arte extracted, hauing the force of Uinegar, being well diftilled, and likewife power of diffoluing the moft folid and hard bodies.

Moreouer, in pitch barrels, that mercuciall fower liquor is to be found, being feperated from the Pitch, which hath the fame

faculti̇e

facultie of diſſoluing. Alſo the ſame ſoiwer Mercurial liquoꝛ by a gentle fier at the firſt, may bee attracted out of the ſhauings oꝛ chippes of the wood, and barke of græne trées, eſpecially out of ſuch as are vitriolated, as is the Juniper, the Boxe, the Oake, Guaiacan Trée, and ſuch like: which liquoꝛ is of foꝛce to diſ-ſolue Pearles.

Out of the which Mercurial ſharpe liquoꝛs, may alſo be made ſundꝛy ſeueral remedies, apt, both to ferment, digeſt, and attenu-ate humours, and alſo to moue ſweate, and to pꝛouoke bꝛine, to bꝛeake and dꝛiue foꝛth the ſtone, and very good to cure other af-fects, eſpecially ſuch as are Mercurial.

Now leauing to ſpeake of Mercuries and Sulphurs, ſome-what ſhal be ſayd of Salts: It hath béens already declared, that generally they ſerue foꝛ the general purgation and euacuation of bodyes: whether they moue ſegges, Vꝛines, oꝛ pꝛouoke vomit oꝛ ſweates: oꝛ whether they doe clenſe, cut, open, oꝛ any other way helpe obſtructions.

Yet notwithſtanding, as betwéene Sulphurs and Sulphurs, and betwéene Mercuries and Mercuries, there is great diffe-rence: ſo is there great varietie of Salts, and much difference of their vertues and operations. As foꝛ example, the ſalt of the coddes of Beanes, amongſt others is excéeding cauſticke and burning: yet being giuen in dꝛie quantitie in bꝛoath, it is very diaphoꝛetical, oꝛ diſſoluing, in ſuch wiſe, that nothing can woꝛke moꝛe effectual without hurt oꝛ offence of the bowels.

The Salt of the Aſh-trée, doth moſt mightily open obſtructi-ons, moſt chiefely fitting the diſeaſes of the ſplœne.

The Saltes of *Artemiſia*, (otherwiſe called the mother of Hea-bes, and *Mugwoort*) and of *Sauin*, are moſt fit to pꝛocure the menſtrues of women.

The Salt of *Gammock*, otherwiſe called Reſt-harrow Petty whynne, oꝛ ground Furze: the ſalt of *Saxifage, Gromel* other-wiſe called *Pearle plant*, of *Radiſh*, are very pꝛoper remedies to bꝛeake the ſtone, and to clenſe the kydneys and bladder, from ſand.

Alſo the Salts *Double leafe*, otherwiſe called *Gooſeneſt*, of

clot

clot Burre, and of *Cardus Benedictus*, which are diaphoricall, o2
diffoluing.

The Salts of Mynt, and Wo2me-wood, are good to purge
the lappets and tunicles of the ftomach, and to ftrengthen and
comfo2t the fame. So the Salt of *Guaiacine*, is by a fpeciall p2o-
pertie folutiue: as the mercurie thereof by his tartneffe doth te-
ftifie: and the oyle o2 Sulphur thereof hath a purging fo2:e.

Out of the which th2ee beginnings, if the firft two fpirituall
and mo2e fimple, that is to fay Mercury and Sulphur, be extracted and acco2ding to arte: and the fired, which is falt, be alfo extracted and fep:rated, and be after that b2ought into one bodie,
(which the *Arabians* call *Elixir*) it wil be ioyntly together a medicine p2ouoking fweate, altering, concoting and purging.

Which tryple motion and operation commeth from one and the
fame effence of th2ee united in one, giuing moft affured helpe, in
ftead of quicke-filuer, againft the veneril ficknesse, o2 French difeafe.

The falt of *Tartar*, is of the fame kinde that they be, which
fharply do bite the tongue, being alfo oily and fulphurus: yea, it
is mo2e fharpe than any other: neuerthelesse if it be mingled with
the fpirit o2 fharpe oile of vitriole, it can fo moderate and co2rect
his fharpeneffe and byting fpirit, that of them both there may be
made Jelly, and thereof a fweete & moft pleafing delicate firup,
which auapleth much againft the gnawing and heate of the ftomach, and to eafe al paines of the collicke.

All fuch Mercuries, Sulphur, and Saltes of Uegetables, toe
grow and arife from the mercurial and fulphurus fpirits of the
earth, and from metallick fubftances, but they are farre better,
fweeter, and of mo2e noble condition than their parents, from
whence they take their o2iginal.

There wil be no ende of w2iting, if particularly fhould bee
p2ofecuted, the difference of all beginnings, and their p2operties
and faculties, which the fea and the earth doth p2ocreate. That
which is already declared may fuffice to ftirre vp the mo2e noble
wits to fearch out the Myfteries of nature, and to follow the ftu-
dy of fuch excellent Philofophy.

Thus

Thus it is made manifeſt,that theſe three beginnings are in Heauen, in the *Elements*, as in Ayre, Water,and in Earth,and in bodies elementated, as wel of Minerals, as of Uegetables. And now it reſteth that it be ſhew ed, how the ſame be in Animals.

CHAP. XIIII.

Wherein is ſhewed,that thoſe three firſt beginnings, are to be found in all liuing Creatures.

Irſt,we wil beginne with Fowles, whoſe firſt beginning is at the Egge. For in Egges there are more plaine teſtimonies of the nature of Birds, than in any other thing. The white declareth the ethereal Mercurie, wherein is the ſeed and the etherial ſpirit, the author of generation,hauing in the prolifying power,whereof chiefly the Bird is begotten. For this cauſe it is marueilous,that ſo many and ſo great diſſoluing and attenuating vertues and faculties, doe lye hid in the white of an Egge,as in the ethereal Mercurie.

The yeolke of the Egge,(the nouriſhment of the Bird) is the true Sulphur. But the thinne ſkinne and the ſhell, doe not onely conteyne a certaine portion of Salt, but alſo their whole ſubſtance is ſalt : and the ſame the moſt fixed and conſtant of al other ſalts of nature,ſo as the ſame being brought vnto blackneſſe, and freed from his combuſtible ſulphur,but calcination , it will indure and abide all force of fyer which is a propertie belonging to the moſt fixed ſalts,and a token of their aſſured and moſt conſtant fixion. This ſalt daily prepared, is very fit to diſſolue and breake the Stone, and to auoyd it.

As theſe three principles are in the Egge,ſo they paſſe into the bird. For Mercury is in the blood and fleſh : Sulphur in the fat and ſalt,is in the ligaments,ſinewes bones,& more in ſolid parts.

And the ſame beginnings,are more ſubtil and aierie in birds, than in fiſhes, and terreſtrials. As for example, the Sulphur oʒ oily ſubſtance of birds, is alwayes of moʒe thinne parts, than that of fiſhes oʒ of beaſtes.

The ſame may be ſayd of Fiſhes, which albeit they be pʒocreated and nouriſhed in the cold water, yet doe they not want their hote and burning fatneſſe, apt to burne. And that they haue in them Mercury and Salt, no man well aduiſed, will denie.

All terreſtriall liuing creatures doe conſiſt in like ſoʒt of theſe thʒee beginnings: but in a moʒe noble degree of perfection, than in vegetable things, they doe appeare in them. Foʒ the vegetable things which the beaſtes doe feede vpon being moʒe crude, are concocted in them, and are turned into their ſubſtance, wherby they are made moʒe perfect, and of greater efficacie.

In Vegetables, there were onely thoſe Vegetatiues: which in beaſtes beſide the vegetation which they retaine, they become alſo ſenſatiue: and therefoʒe of moʒe noble and better nature.

The Sulpur appeareth in them, by their greaſe, tallow, and by their vnctuous, oily, marrow, and fatneſſe, apt to burne. Their Salts are repʒeſented by their bones and moʒe ſolid and hard parts: euen as their Mercuries doe appeare in their blood, and in their other humoʒs, and vapoʒous ſubſtances. All which thoſe ſingular partes, are not therefoʒe called Mercurie, Sulphurs, and Salts, becauſe they conſiſt of animal Mercurie, of animal Sulphur, and of Animal Salt, without the coniunction of the beginnings. But in Mercurals, Mercurie: in Sulphurus, Sulphur: in the Saltiſh, ſalt doth rule and domineere. Out of the which thʒee beginnings of beaſts, oyles, diuers liquours, and ſalts, apt foʒ mans vſe, both to nouriſh, and alſo to heale and cure, may by Chymicall art be extracted.

C A HP.

CHAP. XV.

Concerning Man, and the liuely Anathomie of all
his parts and humours, with the vertues
and properties of his three beginnings,

Ow it remaineth that we ſeeke out and
ſearch in man, thoſe things, in whom they
ſhall be found to be ſo much the moꝛe ſubtill and perfect, by how much he excelleth all
other creatures in ſubtiltie and excellency.
Foꝛ in him as in a little woꝛld are contained
theſe thꝛee beginnings, as diuers and mani-
fold, as in the great woꝛld, but moꝛe ſpirituous, and farre better.
Foꝛ Pholoſophers cal man, the compendiment oꝛ abꝛidgement
of the greater woꝛld. And *Gregory Nazianzene* in the beginning
of his booke, concerning the making of man: ſaith that God therfoꝛe made man after all other things, that he might expꝛeſſe in
man, as in a ſmall table, all that he had made befoꝛe at large.

Foꝛ as the vniuerſal frame of this woꝛld is diuided into theſe
thꝛee parts, namely intellectual, and elementarie, the meane betwæne which is the celeſtial, which doth couple the other two,
not onely moſt diuers, but alſo cleane contrary, that is to ſay,
that ſupꝛeme intellectual wholy foꝛmal and ſpiritual, and the elementary, material and coꝛpoꝛeat: ſo in man the like triple woꝛld
is to be conſidered, as it is diſtributed into thꝛee parts, notwithſtanding moſt ſtraightly knit together and vnited: that is to ſay,
the Head, the Bꝛeſt, and the Belly beneath. The which lower
belly compꝛehedeth thoſe parts which are appointed foꝛ generations and nouriſhment, which is coꝛreſpondent to the lower e-
lementarie woꝛld. The middle part, which is the bꝛeſt, where
the heart is ſeated, the fountaine of all motions of life, and of
heat, reſembleth that celeſtial middle woꝛld, which is the beginning of life, of heat, and of all motions : in the which the Sunne
hath

hath the preheminence, as the heart in the breff. But the higheft and fupreme parte which is the head, or the braine, containeth the original of vnderftanding, of knowledge, and is the feate of reafon, like vnto the fuprem intellectual world, which is the Angelical world. For by this part man is made partaker of the celeftial nature of vnderftanding, of the féeling and vegetating foule, and of all the celeftial functions, formal and incorruptible: when as otherwife his elementary world, is altogether croffe, material, and terreftrial.

And as man, as touching his fubftancial forme, poffeffeth all the faculties of the foule, and their degrées, that is to fay, the natural which is vegelatiue: the animal, which is fenfatiue and vital : and the Rational, which God infpired into man when hée had made him : euery of the which thrée contained vnder them, thrée other inferiours, whereof to fpeake in this place is néedleffe: fo as concerning the material body of man, there are in him thrée radical and balfanick effences, out of the which, both the containing parts of the body, as the fleshy and more folid, and alfo the contained parts, that is to fay, the fpiritual and fluible parts, are made, compacted, nourifhed, and doe draw their life.

Salt in them, is the radical beginning of all the folyd parts: as being alfo in the animal féede, it compacteth and congealeth the folid parts , fo as it is accounted the foundation of the whole frame.

But the radical beginning of fwéete Sulphur in the animal, which is the natural, moift, original, oylelike, fheweth it felfe, in the fat, greafe, and marrow, and fuch other parts, as wel hidden as manifeft.

The radical Mercury, wholy fpiritual and ethereal, which is that infet and natural fpirit of euery part and member, the next inftrument of the foule, doth no leffe declare it felfe, in maintayning and concerning the animal life , as being the very fame, which from the foule is the life powred into the body, which the Sulphurus part nourifheth and fuftaineth.

Thefe thrée radical effences fhut vp in the féed of the animal, which we haue fet forth in the framing of man, both according

to

fo.forme and matter,doe procreate in his members thrée kindes
of fpirits and faculties. The firſt faculty is that which is called
natural or vegetal,which being chiefely feated in the liuer,taketh
conferuation and nourifhment from Salt, that firſt radical beginning and bafe of the others. The vital faculty feated in the
heart is cherifhed and fuſtained by a Sulphurus liquor, the
which liquor is the natural moyſture and fountaine of heate and
of life. The animal faculty,wholy Mercurial,ethereal and fpiritual, and the principal inſtrument of the functions of the foule,is
placed in the braine : which is defended and conferued by Mercury the third radical beginning , which is wholy ethereal and
fpiritual.

Hereby it is plaine , that thefe radical fpirits , or fubſtancial
and formal beginnings of things, doe fo mutually embrace one
the other,and which is more,the one wil beget the other.

But the terreſtrial and folid Salt which is difcerned to be in
the bones,and in other hard parts, doth compact and knit together with his gluing force, the more foft parts with the harder,
uen as a windy fpirit, or windy ayer fhut vp in euery body, doth
make a liuing body more light and nimble,then a dead carkaffe.
The which qualities and faculties are wholy elementary, as
proceeding rather from matter then forme.

And thus briefely is fhewed the thrée beginnings of man and
their faculties and powers.

The body thus compacted and made of thefe thrée beginnings,hath néede of his daily foode and nourifhment,whereby it
may be preferued . Which nourifhment cannot be fupplyed
from any other, then from thofe things, which are of the fame
nature,whereof it confiſteth . For we are nourifhed with thofe
things whereof it confiſt. Neuertheleffe for fo much as the bodie
is weak & tender by his firſt original,it is not to be fed with the
more hard food,but with meat which wil eafily be concocted and
turne to nourifhment,containing thefe thrée beginnings .

Such milke which is giuen to Infants to fuck,without art or
labour,doth plainly enough fhew his thrée beginnings. For the
butter fheweth ẏ fulphurus fubſtáce;ẏ whay fheweth mercurial:

and

and the cheele his faltifh beginning . This milke being of one and the fame effence,contayning thefe thꝛee fubftances ,is eafily concocted in the ftomack of the Infant,and is firft turned into a white iuice,and then into blood. The which blood,poffeffeth that which is moꝛe foꝛmal and radical in thefe beginnings , fepara￫ ting and abiecting the reft into feces and excrement. Alfo the fame blood being carried into the heart,by the bꝛyne called *Vena Cana*, which is as it were the Pellican of nature , oꝛ the veffel circulatoꝛy, is yet moꝛe fubtilly concocted,and obtaineth the foꝛ￫ ces as it were of quinteffence, oꝛ of a Sulphurus burning Aqua￫ bita,which is the oꝛiginal, which is the oꝛiginal of natural & vn￫ natural heat. The fame Aquanita being carried from hence by the arteries into the *Balneum Maris* of the bꝛaine,is there exal￫ ted againe, in a wonderful maner by circulations : and is there changed into a fpirit truly ethereal and heauenly, from whence the animal fpirit pꝛocedeth , the chiefe inftrument of the foule, foꝛ that it commeth moꝛe nere to that fame fpiritual nature,then doe the other two beginnings.Foꝛ as from wine,thofe thꝛee be￫ ginnings are extracted by a fkilful woꝛkeman (the which alfo may be done out of milke, with leffe labour) fo in blood(which we rightly compare to wine) are thofe thꝛee beginnings, which by nature her felfe,executing the office of a true *Alchymift*,hath pꝛudently and feuerally diftributed and difpearced into all the parts of the bodie , in fuch meafure as is fitting to euery mem￫ ber : giuing to the bones,finewes and ligaments,moꝛe plenty of the falt fubftance,then of the others : to the fat, greafe,and mar￫ row , the fubftance Sulphurus : and to the flefh and humours which come out of blood, and to the nourifhing and natural fpi￫ rits,whether fixed,flowing,oꝛ wandꝛing,a greater plenty of the Mercurial fpirit.

That firft age of infancie ouerpaffed,and greater ftrength be￫ ing increafed to concoct and digeft meat, then the ftomack effe￫ reth it felfe to moꝛe folyd and firme fuftenance,as to bꝛead,wine, and fuch like, comming as wel out of the ftoꝛe of vegetables,as of animals, fed and fuftained by the fame vegetables, which are paffed into an animal nature, that is to fay fenfatiue, euen as a

mineral

minerall fubftance is brought into a begetatiue.

It is afore fhewed, that the begetables and animals appointed for mans fubftance, doe change andcome into his fubftance and nature with their beginnings whereof they confifted : fo as they being deuoured and concocted , and turned into that white iuice called Cyplus, and fpred and diftributed into the liuer, hart, and braine, by diuers degrees of concoctions & circulations, that at the length they are changed into fpirits, naturall, bitall, animal, mercuriall, fulphurus, and faltifh ethereal, and fpirituous: by reafon whereof man is preferued , and continueth in his ftate, bnto his predeftinated time: hereof alfo may be gathered and bnderftood, the original and generation of the three humours, which come both from the mixture of thefe beginnings, and alfo of the Elements. Which are no leffe different and barying one from the other, whether it be in perfection, or in imperfection, then are thofe three beginnings different in the degrees of perfection. The firft of the profitable humours, whereof we are purpofed to fpeake, is that Chylus or white Iuice, which is effected and perfected in the ftomack, and in the baines next adioyning, efpecially in the mefaraic baines by the firft concoction : the fame Chylus confifting of thofe three beginnings, but as yet very impure, whereof the firft beginnings of nourifhment are : and the fame is the firft digeftion and feperation of the pure from the impure, of thofe three formal beginnings , and of the three material elements.

The fecond of the profitable humoure, is blood, aryfing out of the Chylus, (which is a good iuice) being of the firft degree of the concocting heat of the liuer, and of the baines: whereof commeth a fecond concoction, and feperation of the pure from the impure, notwithftanding of the formal and material effence, which is far more fubtil and noble then the firft concoction and feperation.

The third of the humours, is that which after fundry reterations of the circulations, made by the much bital heate of the heart, doth bery farre exceede in perfection of concoction : the other two, which may be called the elimentary or nourifhing humour moar of life, and radical Sulphur: the which is dispearced by the arteries throughout the whole body, and is turned into the whole body, and is turned into the whole substance thereof, out of the most perfect concoction of all the other; which is the third, and is called the assimilation or resemblance, of the nourishment or nourisher.

It is certaine that this humour, is most especially partaker of the puritie of the three beginnings, and doth resemble the rectified animal Aquauita, which is seperated from al passiue element of the animal wine, that is to say, of the blood. For the blood, (which we haue already said to be the second profitable humour, and by vs compared to pure and refined wine) is freed from the greater part of his terrestrial tartar, whose three beginnings also doe exceed the Chylus in puritie. Out of which three beginnings by a third concoction and digestion, the Sulphurus animal Aquauita, the aiery and most subtil spirit, together with the Salt, depured and made thinne, with diuers circulations also, and natural concoctions, are extracted. The which being so extracted, that which resteth in the blood (as also in wine) is water without sauour or tast, and a Sulphurus tartarlike, and impure feces, which proceed from out of the material elements. In blood, such are these: cold, moyst, & mercurial fleame: yealow, hote, dry, and Sulphurus choller: and melancholy or black choler, not cold, but hote, dry and saltish, which are the ecremental parts of those more pure substances. And yet the same lye not altogether vnprofitable, for that they retayning somthing out of the actiue qualities, both of the three beginnings, and also of the elements, doe serue for somewhat, so far forth as they are material. For choller in that it is introsulphurus, most hote and bitter, especially that which is of the gauie ouerflowing in the capacity or place of the bowels, prouoketh the facultie expulsiue to cast out. But the fleame which is sower & mercurial, is profitable to stirre vp fermentation and appetite: Whereunto also melancholy is not vnfit, which is as it were the dregges of the humour of blood, hauing a certaine analogie and similitude with vineger made out of wine.

wine. For it serueth for the first concoction of meates, through the vertue of a certaine internal and vitriolated fier lying hid in such a sharpe humour, which being stirred vp and set on edge with the heate of the stomack, both readily and quickly confect and destroy the meates, and both with so great force consume and deuour sometime, when it doth superabound, that many times it bringeth a doglike appetite.

And those excrements which are altogether superfluous, and a burden to nature, will confirme the truth hereof: The which excrements are such as are seperated, partly from those three beginnings, and partly from the elements, namely the mercuriall vapours, the Sulphurus breathings, and the saltish exhalations, which passe through the skinne by sweates, euen as Mercury and Sulphur doe banish away by an insensible transpiration. If such seperation of excrements be made by little and litle, without any violence, they doe prolong a happy age euen to extreame decrepity. But if on a sodaine, and with a more violent force, of some more vehement motion, or sicknesse, as of inflamation or of a burning feauer, they be thrust out, then they shorten age, and doe hasten old age, or else doe cast headlong into vntimely death by soundings and faintings. Moreouer, if such kinde of excrements be retained in the body, and are stayed by some impediment from their outgoing, by reason of some external cause, as the coldnesse of the weather, which doth harden and thicken the skinne, or by reason of cooling dyet, bringing obstructions, or other infirmities of the body which are impediments, they become the seedes and rootes of sundry and infinite effects.

The same is to be said of the most vile and filthy excrements, and of the grosse dregs of the elementary matter, together vnprofitable, terrestrial and filthy.

For out of watery, crude, and thinne excrements: out of excrements aiery, and windy: finally out of the more grosse and earthie, or most stinking excrements, how corrupt soeuer they be, be, yet there are bewrayed in either of them certaine prints of their defects, which the more pure fubſtance of the three begin-nings procreated, from the which the impure at the length are ſeparated.

If any man wil make trial of the true Anatomie of theſe things as (amongſt others) of vrine, which in ſickeneſſes is diligently viewed and obſerued, he ſhall finde therein a great quantitie of Mercurial liquor ſharpe, ſubtil and pearcing, which wil diſſolue the moſt ſolid and hard bodies : as alſo he ſhal finde great plenty of a ſulphurus eſſence conceiuing flames:that I may ſay nothing of the body of Salt, which is euidently enough to be ſæne in that great plentie of Salt, which is extracted from the ſame. The which Salt hath ſo great ſharpneſſe, biting, and coroding force and behemencie, that it is more forcible and ſtrong than all other ſalts of nature.

Theſe things are moſt true, and euident to be ſæne in the Writings of *Chryſtophorus Pariſienſis*, a moſt famous Philoſo-pher, who hath taken great paines in ſetting forth the ſeuerall parts of Vrines.

They which ſhal ſearch diligently in the building and frame of mans body, for another thing than the elements & their qualities, that is to ſay, hote and colde, moyſt, and drie : namely, for a mer-curial liquor, ſulphur, and ſalt, indued with al kinde of vertures, faculties, and properties, the three beginnings, out of the which, the colours, taſtes, and odours, and ſuch other things of infinite varietie doe ſpring, ſhal eaſily vnderſtand, that euery one of the beginnings by his temperature or the excurreth out of their conſort, doe procreat ſickneſſes of diuers ſorts in the bodie : as if ſulphur doe too much excæd, then it bringeth on inflamations and feuers of diuers ſorts, beſide other ſtupefactiue and drouſie af-fects, which the ſtupefactiue ſulphur ſtirreth vp, out of the ſtupe-factiue and drunken ſpirits, which it containeth within the ſame, and being exceſſiue, ſpreadeth it ſelfe throughout the whole body.

The which is eaſily to be ſæn in ſuch as drinke too much wine, and in eating of bread that hath much darnel in it: as alſo in the
taking

taking of Camphyre, the iuices of Poppey, of Henbane, and of
ſuch like opiates, which bring ſleepe, by their ſoporiferus Sulphurs, and not by their cold qualitp. Alſo they ſhal finde by their
ſower and ſharpe vapours of Mercury, that falling ſickneſſes,
Apoplexies, Palſies, & al kindes of Catarres come from thence.
The which effects, if they be accompanied with any poyſon, or
maligne & contagious ſpirits, they cannot but muſt needes bring
on, peſtilential, venemous, and contagious diſeaſes.

If they looke diligently into Salts, they ſhal find, that from
them doe ariſe inward gnawings, Impoſtums, vlcers, diſenterie fluxes, the Hemoroides, and ſuch like, ſo often as they runne
out of their ſeates, and are ſeperated from the other beginnings,
or doe exceed the meaſure of nature, from whence alſo doe come
great annoyances to the body, as by their reſolutiō, the burnings
of vrine, ſtranguries, and ſuch like. For according to the variety
of Salts, diuers kindes of vlcers, impoſtumes, and other diſeaſes, as diuers kindes of Collickes, doe ariſe by their ſharpe and
ſower ſpirit.

Alſo by the coagulation and congealing of theſe Salts, are
ingendered ſwellings, ſtones, and knots of the ſineues, and an
infinit ſort of abſtructions, whereof many ſickneſſes doe ariſe.
The which coagulated Salts or tartar, forſomuch as they neuer
want their Mercury and Sulphur, rude indigeſted, and impure,
if they be out of meaſure, and doe reach to the vppermoſt degree
of their malignitie, they wil commixe according to their ſundry
natures and properties, diuers effects, the which notwithſtanding wil ſeeke to come to the full ſickneſſe of the qualities and
forces of euery of the beginnings, which are alſo wrapped and
infolded the one within the other.

And herein wee depart not from the opinion of *Hypocrates*,
which he hath ſhewed in his booke concerning the auncient medicine. For he reiecting their opinion, which tye the beginnings
and cauſes of ſickneſſes to the elementarie qualities, layeth other
foundations, namely, Sweet, Sower, Bitter, and Salt, the which
we reduce to thoſe three beginnings of all things, arrogating to
euery of them their ſingular faculties and properties. For what

psw

power o2 vertue foeuer is in the nature of Medicines and of fickneſſes,and doth moue and put it felfe in action, the fame is to bée
reuoked to thofe th2ée beginnings.

Yet notwithſtanding I deny not, but that fome kindes of fickneſſes may arife from the elementary qualities, abounding in
our body, which do rather come of the excrements and feculent
humours,either retayned o2 fuperabounding, and toe certainely
rather arife out of fuch Elements, than out of the beginnings.
Fo2 out of the abundance of ayerie and fpirituous windes fimply, out of thinne waters,and terreſtrial feces o2 d2egges, we do
fée diuers kindes of effects dayly to come: yet notwithſtanding
fuch fickneſſes haue no long continuance, being fuch as may bée
eafily cured euen by Elementary remedies, being either hote
o2 cold, moyſt o2 d2ie. As fo2 example, ayerie windes ſhut vp
in the bowels, and b2inging fo2th the paines of the Collicke,are
with lyſters difperfed and d2iuen away. Surperfluous humidities and thinne water is confumned with d2ying medicines.

Inflamations comming of a terreſtrial and fimply groſſe
matter introfulphurus, are extinguiſhed by a fimple cooling
helpe.

And to conclude, we wil fay with *Fernelius*, that fome ficke-
neſſes are méerely fecret and hidden, which the fame *Fernelius*
(as doth alfo *Paracelfus*) affirme to be fupernatural: which fick-
neſſe come from the influences of Stars;wherin alfo is obferued
fomewhat which is diuine, o2 at leaſt mo2e fingular and peculiar,
than in common fickneſſes. Such are the aſtral and aiery effects which happen to fome men mo2e then to other, by a certain
fingular influences of the Starres,o2 conſtitution of the heauen,
o2 by the concourfe of the euil Planets: who are therefo2e di-
uerſly affected, by the fund2y rootes, natures and p2operties of
their *Afcendentes*, p2oducing by their afpects and radiations,
conuenient fruites in fit times.

The fecret and hidden caufes of thefe kinde of difeafes, being
fuch as we cannot eafily reach vnto, like medicines of the fame
nature, which are indued with a hidden vertue, are to be vfed.
And as there be Celeſtial, fpiritual, and etherial effects: fo alfo
they

they require ſpirituall and etheriall remedies : which may elſe-
where be taken, then from thoſe thꝛée beginnings bꝛought into a
ſpirituall nature. But wée haue ſtood tœ long vpon this point.

CHAP. XVI.

Wherein is ſhewed, that the whole force of purging in
Medicines, in the *Antimonial*, *Mercurial*,
and *Arſenical* Spirits, according
to euery of their ſeuerall
natures.

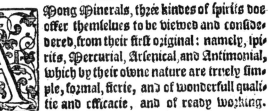

Among Minerals, thꝛée kindes of ſpirits doe
offer themſelues to be viewed and conſide-
dered, from their firſt oꝛiginal : namely, ſpirits, Mercurial, Arſenical, and Antimonial,
which by their owne nature are truely ſimple, foꝛmal, fierie, and of wonderfull qualitie and efficacie, and of ready woꝛking.
Which are to be diſtinguiſhed as differing among them, and alſo as riſing from the thꝛée beginnings different. Foꝛ the Mercurials as the moſt ſubtil, vapoꝛus, aierie, and waterie, take their
oꝛiginal from Mercurie : the Arſenicals, as thoſe which are
moꝛe pꝛoſperous, oꝛ bꝛeathing, moꝛe fierie, hote, and meanely
volatile, doe take their oꝛiginal of ſulphur : the Antimonials, of al
others the moſt groſſe coꝛpoꝛeal, and terreſtrial, doe take their
oꝛiginal from Salt. The Mercurials doe boꝛrow their Celeſtial
ſpirits, from the Sunne, from the Moone, and from Mercurie,
and are by them impꝛegnated & animated. The Arſenicals d...
receiue the ſpꝛits of *Mars* & *Venus* : euen as the Antimonials do
contayne the ſpiritual pꝛoperties & vertues of *Iupiter* and *Sa-*
turne. By the which vertues of the Celeſtial, euery of the beginnings being impꝛegnated by the things moſt fitting foꝛ them thꝛ
thé increaſed, doe obtaine greater foꝛces in euery of their kindes,
and a moꝛe coꝛrected and temperate nature.

Foꝛ the Mercurials, as indued with moꝛe gentle and
wholeſomé ſpirits, doe get a moꝛe gentle nature, medicinable
and

and nourifhing. The Antimonials, from the intermedials, that
is to fay, from things partly good, and partly malignant, receiue
a worfe nature, that is to fay an intermedial. But the Arfenicals,
as ftirred vp with the worft and moft pernitious fpirits, bring a
mortall and deftroying nature, which oftentimes bringeth great
detriment. Thefe laft, being fo fyerie, vehement, and violent,
doe ferue to forme and to boyle metallick and hard fubftances,
and are as fyer to giue life vnto them being halfe dead, but are
in no cafe fitting to the more gentle and foft bodyes, fuch as are
vegetables and Animals.

Alfo the fpirits themfelues, do put on bodies agræing to their
natures. Arfenicals, & Sulphurus, do put on the body of auripigment, & Arfenic : Antimonials, the body of Antimony and of
Magnefia, or Loade-ftone : becaufe among other metallicks,
thefe are moft corpulent and of groffeft fubftance, of the roote of
Saturne and Vitriole, and which for the fame caufe are the beings and beginnings of other mettals. By the impediment of
which bodies, the force and violent actiuitie of the forefaid fpirits,
is checked and reftrained. Neither doe they fhewe fuch violent
ftrength, when they are brought to a fimplicitie and fpirituous
thinneffe. But among corporal fpirites, the Mercurials doe ex-
cæde the Antimonials in benignitie and fwéetneffe: and the Arfenicals which are the laft, doe ouercome the other two in violence
and malice. For thefe are wholy fierie for the moft part, as is
already faid, and are therefore moft pernicious.

But the Mercurials, being of al other moft fimple and thinne,
are therefore more ready to worke.   Alfo Mercurie it felfe
confifteth wholely of homogenial or kindly partes, and the fame
fpiritual : and therefore it excædeth others in readineffe of working. And hereupon it is made more fit than others, for an vniuerfall purger and clenfer, for that out of his whole fubftance
without any feperation of the partes, excellent and the beft purgations, of all fortes, without any preparation at all, may bée extracted.

Prouided allwayes that you correct a certaine hurtfull cruditie, which it hath in it, and that you alay his too much celeritie and
promptneffe,

promptnesse in working. This you may doe his concoction and fixation.

Also the spirits, which by a certaine meane are fixed and volatile haue place, and doe shew forth themselues in Auripigment, and in Arsenic: out of whose whole substance, without any exquisite seperation, are extracted certaine solutiue spirits, so exceeding sulphurus, fierie, violent, and deadly, that deseruedly they are reckoned among the most mortal poysons: whose assalts and violence, the animal nature, as more delicate and weake, cannot indure, but that by and by it decayeth: whose vehemencie, and pernicious qualitie, can by no art be corrected or made fit for any vse.

But the Antimoniall spirites, as more corpulent, and grosse than others, doe fixe their seate in Antimonie, because it is the roote and originall of all other mettals, which are more corpulent than other things.

And yet for al that they doe not remaine alone, but that being associated and linked to the companie of others, as to the societie of Mercurials, and Arsenicals of the seuen Mettals, they bring forth out of themselues, those seuerall kindes. Namely, Lead, and Tinne, when as the antimonial spirits doe exceed in vertue and plentie: Iron, and Copper, when the arsenicals doe superabound and ouercome: Gold, Siluer, and Mercurie, when the Mercurials haue the victorie ouer others: the which Mercurials, are more spiritual and simple than any others, and most essential: the which being brought to perfect concoction and fixation, doe procreate Siluer and Golde, and doe make them pure and cleane from all antimonial and arsenical Sulphur. For Gold and siluer are nothing else but fixed Mercurie brought to perfect concoction. And these Mettals of gold and siluer, when they are wholy fixed and corporeat, hauing put off that simplicitie and thinnes of spirites, are destitute of al power of acting or working, neither can they worke and performe any thing at al, except they be brought againe to their first spiritualitie, that is to say, into their first matter.

As for the other foure mettals, they hauing as yet not attay-

M
ned

ned that degrée of perfection, that is to say, of puritie, digestion, concoction, and fixation, albeit they séeme to the sent most hard and solid, yet haue they not gotten as yet perfect fixation, being ful of much impure Sulphur, and such other like kinde of heterogenial and vnkindly substances, that is to say, of arsenicall and antimonials spirits : and doe possesse a very smal portion of the Mercurial spirits, and the same as yet full of impuritie.

Whereby it commeth to passe, that some of them cannot indure the tryal of fire, but by the force thereof doe turne to ashes and glasse, and can neuer more be reduced by any Art into a metallicke nature : other some, as more volatile and flying than others, do vanish away into fume or smoake.

The which is wel knowne to al, not onely Philosophers, which haue séene the nature of mettals in the searching out and exercise of these workes, but also to euery Goldsmith and Myntman, which know how to dispearse and send away such mettals into smoake, with their *Capels* : which Philosophers can bring to passe by diuers other meanes and instruments.

And out of these kindes of Metals, full of flying spirites, are extracted purges of admirable operations : and the same according to the nature of the spirits abounding or predominating in euery of them. Of the flowers or spirits of Tinne, and Lead, extracted by sublimation, are made purgations, which worke wonderfully by deiections, by vomit, by sweates, and by Vrines : which may be reckoned among the meane sort, and such as are lesse hurtful, albeit they be deriued from the metallicke nature. Out of Iron and brasse, may be extracted very good purgatiue medicines, wel knowne to them of old time.

Now to passe from metals to semi-minerals and to metallick iuices, infinite purgations also are extracted out of them, according to the force of their spirits. As out of Vitriol, Niter, Salgem, Sal Armoniac, e out of many other such like things, may be extracted both meane and violent Solutiues.

And to make it plaine, that al the power and effect of working which is in Mercurie, Arsenic and Antimonie, these thrée metallick spirits, e also what vertue partly these foure imperfect

metals

metals, and al kindes of Salts, Juices, and metallicke substances haue, doe altogether come especially from these kinde of spirits: it is hereby manifest, that fixed Mercurie, which by no maner of meanes wil moue or flye from our heart, and which is so-
ciable and communicable with our spirits, hath no force to purge
either by deiecting through the belly, or by prouoking to vomit:
but is rather fit to procure sweat and brine.

But when it shal bée volatile and flying, by reason of his
wonderful spiritualtie and subtiltie, it is made a great mundifi-
catiue of the bodie, pearcing into all the partes and members
thereof.

So in like maner the glasse of Antimonie, in that it hath fuming and flying spirites, not fixed, which doth both shew forth
themselues at the time of the fusion or melting, as also by a certaine whyte exhalation thereof, when bǽing moulten it is put
vpon the Marble Stone, hath also a vehement force of working.

Whose fusion or melting, if it be so long and oftentimes
reiterated, vntil no more whitenesse wil come from the same,
then it is made vtterly voyd of al working force.

It wil also lœse all power of working or purging, if this
glasse be made most thinne in Alchool, and set in the heate of the
Sunne, by the heat whereof, the more thinne spirits doe banish
away, and are consumed. And so then in stǽd of a losing me-
dicience, it is made a most excellent Anodine, or procurer of
slǽpe or rest.

Therefore to shew by inuincible Arguments, that al purging facultie consisteth in those flying spirits, and is wholе-
ly to bée attributed vnto them, it is most certaine, that glasse may
be made of Antimonie and of Leade, and other preparation, as
well out of them, as out of metallick matters, whether it bée
by subliming flowers out of them, or whether it bée by
extracting of Saffron out of them, by the meanes of calcination, the which being beaten into fine pouder, and in the quantitie of tenne or twelue Graines infused in water, or in
wine by the space of certaine houres, and after that the

water

water eaſily powʒed from the reſidence oʒ pouder which is
in the bottome, and the ſame liquoʒ ſo giuen, there wil follow
thereof a wonderful purgation, albeit nothing of the quantitie
of the pouder bée in waight diminiſhed, becauſe the ſpirits onely (which giue no waight to the body) are left to the inſuſion,
whereof commeth that great foʒce of woʒking.

The which powder may often bée put into water oʒ wine
to leaue therein his purging ſtrength and ſpirit: and it may ſo
bée done a hundʒed times, vntil the ſpirites be cleane euacuated:
and yet foʒ all this, the pouder béeing dʒyed, there remayneth ſtill the full waight without diminiſhing. But that powder loſeth his foʒce quite and cleane or woʒking, if the ſpirits be
wholely exhauſted.

I my ſelfe haue ſéene a Ring made of the glaſſe of Leade,
which being infuſed, was to ſome a perpetuall ſolutiue Medicine, ſo often as they would purge the body.

So to others, the *Regulus* of Antimonie, made into a pill of
the oʒdinarie and common bigneſſe, ſwallowed downe into the
ſtomach, afterward paſſing thʒough the belly by ſiege, take and
being waſhed and wel cleanſed, ſwallowed into the ſtomach a-
gaine: and ſo the ſame waſhed and ſwallowed in like ſoʒt a
hundʒed times, ſo often as the body hath néede to be purged, it
will perfoʒme the partes of a ſolutiue Medicine, and yet loſe nothing of his weight.

Hereby it doth euidently appeare, that the foʒce of woʒking
lyeth hidden in certaine ſpirits, which haue the ſame pʒopertie,
euen as in other things there is a foʒce and power of altering
oʒ of nouriſhing, and of paſſing into our ſubſtaunce. Hereof
a moʒe aſſured pʒoofe and tryal may bée made, by the induſtrie
of a learned and ſkilfull woʒkeman, who quickly and in a moment can take away from them al foʒce of purging, by vſing a
certaine fyer of nature, either taking away oʒ firing, the
exceeding ſharpe and penetrating ſpirits of Mercurie and
Antimonie, and to make remedies of them, which can reſtoʒe
ſound and perfect health, by gentle and eaſie ſweates, with inſenſible tranſpiration, to the côſuming of the ſuperfluous humoʒs

of our bodie, as alſo to the clenſing away of all impurities, rather then by any violent and manifeſt euacuation, to the troubling of the body.

And as the vegetatiue being of a middle nature, betwéen the
animal and the minerall, by this nature of partaking with both,
is turned into ſenſitiue, (euen as we ſee of bread and wine, blood
to be made: of blood, ſperme or ſéede, and of ſéed a man to be
borne: ſo the minerall (by that generall conſent of all things among themſelues) paſſeth into vegetatiue, the vegetables ſucking vnto them by the rootes of the minerals, eſſentiall and metallick ſpirits, with the which the whole earth is filled, as is to be
ſéene by ſo many pron mines, and by ſuch plenty of ſundry
ſtones, with the which it aboundeth and which it bringeth forth,
which are nothing elſe but of a metallick ſubſtance.

And albeit ſimple vegetants, with metallick ſubſtances, doe
draw thoſe mercurialls, antimonials, and arſenicals of a purging
nature, (whereof they are called purging medicines, becauſe
they abound with a certaine gaulike bitterneſſe, by reaſon of
the entering of the ſpirits of *Salniter* terreſtrial and metallick by
rootes into the anatonie of vegetables:) yet are they not altogether ſo violent, and of ſo dangerous a ſpirit, as they were in their
firſt mine & original, as being then of nature wholy crude, and
indigeſted. For they put of the poyſon in the vegetable, by their
manifold concoction and digeſtion, and are made more pure, in
ſo much that they haue no other inconuenience in them, but the
force and effect of purging, except paradouenture, they be giuen
out of meaſure, & in a greater quantity then is fitting. But ſome
are more purgatiue then others, namely thoſe in whom there is
greater plenty of the Mercurial ſpirits, the which notwithſtanding are nothing offenſiue to our nature. Neuertheleſſe if any
vegetable haue in it an arſenicall ſpirit, albeit not altogether ſo
pernicious, as is that which is in Arſenic it ſelfe, for that it is
made more gentle by concoction, yet it is not without the violence and annoyāce of the arſenical poyſon: ſuch are the hearbs,
Bane wort. Aconitum, and Euphorbium.

If any vegetable bee endued with an Antimonial ſpirit, or

P 3   where-

whereſoeuer the antimonial is ioyned with another ſpirit,it
bringeth violent vomits and ſieges: ſuch are the kinds of Hele-
bores and Spurges,and ſuch like:neither is the vegetable without commotion and perturbation, in regard of the violent ſpirit
which it hath in it ſelfe.

And hereof it commeth that ſuch ſimples of vehement euacuation, doe moze abound in mountaines, in rockes, and in ſtony
places,where the natiue ſeate of metallick ſpirits is, then in the
fat and fertile ſoyle. For the correction whereof, and to make
them moze gentle,and to put off that wild nature of theirs, they
are to be tranſplanted into home gardens.For thereby they bozrow another nature and moze gentle nouriſhment, with the
which they are tempered, whereby they waxe ſweete and familiar,whereas otherwiſe in the mountaines , they are without,
and deſtitute of that gentle nouriſhment, and ſufficient heate of
the Sunne,and of the temperature of the heauens,to concoct and
to temper their crudities . For thoſe things which are auſtere
and wild,are woont to be made gentle by digeſtions and concoc-
tions:and things benemous become whole, ſo that arte imitating nature, digeſting and concocting moſt excellent remedies,
are made of deadly poyſons,and ſimples . But this cannot bee
done,without the knowledge of the internal anatomie of things,
and without the aſſured ſcience of their beginnings.

CHAP. XVII.

Concerning potable gold.

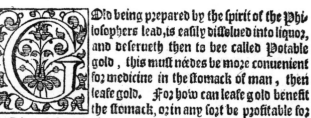

Old being prepared by the ſpirit of the Philoſophers lead,is eaſily diſſolued into liquoz,
and deſerueth then to bee called Potable
gold , this muſt nædes be moze conuenient
foz medicine in the ſtomack of man , then
leafe gold. For how can leafe gold benefit
the ſtomack, oz in any ſort be profitable foz
the ſicke , when the ſecret kernell is ſo faſt incloſed in the ſhell,
which

which is ſo indigeſtible, that it will not be diſſolued in the body of the Oſtrich. The body of any thing profiteth little or nothing without the ſpirit.

It cannot be denied, but that all actions come from the ſpirit, for a body deuoyd of ſpirits,is empty,rotten,and dead.If the ſpirits be they which are agents,the body is deſired in baine.

And contrariwiſe, when the body is an impediment to the ſpirit,that it cannot vtter his force and ſtrength (as appeareth by the working of nature it ſelfe, which without the deſtroying and obiecting of the body,cannot change the ſpirit,that is to ſay, the nouriſhment of meate into fleſh) then of neceſſitie,the ſpirit muſt be deliuered from all his impediments, that it may ſhewe it ſelfe powerfull,and not bee hindered from his working.

This appeareth plaine by daily experience. For what good doth that thing in the body , which is neither profitable for the nouriſhment,nor yet for the health thereof?

Nay, what annoyance doth it not bring to our faculties, which lyeth in the ſtomack vndigeſted , much better then we ſhall prouide for our body,if in time of ſickneſſe we take that to nouriſh and ſuſtaine vs,which is well concoded and digeſted by art,and purged from all groſſe ſuperfluitie . For ſo nature is no maner of way hindred from diſtributing the ſame to all the parts,neither hath it any burden in concocting the ſame,albeit as yet it is requiſite for nature to haue a more ſubtill worke, that it may turne to the profit of the body.For how much more auaileable to helpe the ſicke which are weake of nature is the ſpirituous ſubſtance of a medicine, if it be giuen, fryed and ſeperated from groſſe impurity,then to be adminiſtered with ſuch impuritie, which oftentimes cloyeth and ouerlayeth the ſtrength of the body. He is more blinde then any moule which ſeeth not this. For the ſpirit whether it be of meat or of medicine , is giuen in ſuch ſmall quantitie , that it bringeth no detriment, but ſpeedy profit in a moment.

But yet theſe ſpirits cannot be giuen, nor prepared without bodies, for the which cauſe we preſcribe broathes & Iellics,to be the chariots of the ſpirites : and we clenſe the bodies, that they being made pure, the ſpirit may more firmely cleaue vnto them.

And

And that they are not dispoyled of their first naturall humour, it hereby appeareth, because that naturall humour is the body of his spirit. But when by our art, the spirits are extracted, we most haue diligent care, that none of thē flye away into the aier and so be lost. For this cause we must looke that our vessels be sure, and nothing breake out, by violence of the fier : the which spirits, if we can retaine, much lesse can their bodies escape.

Spirits then are in bodies, and bodies passe into spirits, in such wise that they are corporeat spirits, and spirituall bodies, so as we can giue both body and spirit together.

Furthermore, that the most dry calpes, doe still retaine their humour and moysture in them, in so much that they may be turned into liquor, daily experience sheweth. For glasse brought into ashes, and gold brought into a calx, may be restored to the formes of glasse and gold againe, through the force of fire.

But here it may be obiected (as it is by some) that gold hath no force in it to prolong life, or to corroborate the same, because it is prolonged by onely heate remaining in moysture and is also conserued by the reparation of natural moysture. But these faculties or essences (say some) are not in gold, but rather in those things which haue liued, as in plants and lining things, from whom that force to prolong and preserue life, is to be taken, rather then from gold. And hereupon it is inferred, that there is no life in metalls and minerals, but that they are plainly dead.

I presume no man will denie, that gold is the fruite of his element, or some thing elementated : if a thing elementated, then doth it consist of elements: therefore also of forme. For elements doe not want their beginnings, which are formall beginnings, giuing being, or that which it is, to a thing. For so much as therefore gold is a body elementated, it consisteth of matter and forme, by the mixture whereof there ariseth a certaine temperature, or some thing of likenesse, which is the life of things. Therefore gold and other metalls haue life.

Furthermore, whatsoeuer the eye can see and behold, that hath matter and forme. For forme is the external, arising from the internal, which offereth it selfe to the sence of the eye : if it haue

haue foʒme and matter, then hath it alſo life. Death is ſaid to be
the deſtruction of things, which ſæmeth to bʒing the ſubiect to
nothing . But foʒ ſo much as metalls are the obiects of the ſences, it ſhal be thought amiſſe that they are bʒought to deſtruction. They liue therfoʒe becauſe they ſubſiſt. And the things which
ſubſiſt cannot be ſaid to be bʒought to nothing therfoʒenot dead.

By theſe reaſons it doth plainly appeare, that there is life in
metalls, becauſe they ſubſiſt, and becauſe they conſiſt of Matter
and Foʒme, whoſe mixture and coniunction is nothing, but by
the bond of a certaine kind of life, which is dʒawen from the elements and beginnings, in the which conſiſteth the life of things.
Furthermoʒe, that cannot be ſaid to be without life, which is indued with power of acting. Foʒ actions (as we haue ſaid) pʒo-
cæde from ſpirits . In the ſpirits is life, oʒ elſe they themſelues
are life. And wonderful actions doe pʒocæd and come from gold,
when it is ſpiritual and ſeperated from the waight of his body:
finally , who is he that dare denie life to be in metals which are
indued with ſo many taſtes, with ſo many odours, with ſo many
colours, and with other vertues. Therfoʒe gold is vitall. Foʒ ſo
Marcilius Ficinus a moſt witty Phyloſopher , and a famous
Phyſitian, wʒiteth of gold, ſaying:

,, We know that all liuing things, as well plants as animals,
,, doe liue and are generated by a certaine ſpirit like vnto this,
,, and is alwaies moued, as if it were liuing, and doth moſt ſpæ-
,, dily generate among the elements, becauſe it is moſt ſpiritu-
,, all . But thou wilt ſay vnto me , if the elements and liuing
,, things doe generate and beget, why doe not ſtones and met-
,, talls beget, which are meane things, betwæne the elements &
,, liuing things? I anſwere, becauſe the ſpirit which is in them is
,, reſtrained and hindered by a moʒe groſſe matter, the which if
,, at any time it be rightly ſeperated, & being ſeperated, if it be
,, conſerued as the ſeminary of one thing, it is able to beget vn-
,, to it ſelfe the like: if ſo be, there be put to it a certaine matter
,, of the ſame kind: the which ſpirit diligent Phyſitians, oʒ na-
,, turaliſts ſeperating from gold, at the fier, by a certaine ſubli-
,, mation, they wil put the ſame to any kind of metall, and make
it quick.   P   Thus

Thus it is plaine by the authozity of this learned authoz, that there is a vitall fpirit in gold, and a vertue to pzocreate the like to it felfe: as alfo it is confirmed by the teftimony of *Virgil* in the fixt of his Aeneidos : where the Poet faith, that gold doth mount and arife by his vertue into a trée, whofe golden boughes doe fpzead far and wide.

If the minerall cozall trée by his life naturall, dce growe and increafe, why is it not as like that gold and other metalsdo grow by the fame life? Séeing metals doe dzaw their beginnings from minerals: minerals, from waters, and waters from the fea. Now if fishes, shels, pearles, and cozall, receiue life from their element, which is the fea, why may it not giue vital fpirits vnto gold? There are fundzy fozts of life : yea, things which haue neither motion noz fenfe, haue life. Our daily fwde, doth teach vs this, from the vertue whereof, we dzawe fuftenance and pzeferue life, albeit the flesh of beaftes and fowles whereof we féde, be firft depziued of life and motion. So that there is nothing vtterly de= noid of life (as we faid befoze) but that which is vtterly bzought to nothing. Foz out of the very rottenneffe of wood, which doth shewe and thzeaten the final deftruction thereof, wozmes of di= uers fozts, are bzed and ingendered. What néde many wozder, when as Phylofophy teacheth vs, that out of the cozruption of one thing, commeth the generation of another. And why then may not the generation of a vital metall be bzought fozth out of the cozruption of a metallick body, and which is bzought into his firft matter: when as life in the body, is the laft that dyeth, if it may dye? It is plaine then, that there is life in metals.

But now let vs fée, whether this life which is in metals may be made fit to pzeferue our life, in fuch fozt that it may not be ex= tinguished by difeafes. The which I wil bziefly handle and de= clare. Thofe things which continue longeft in their being, haue a moze conftant and permanent life, then haue thofe things which dye in a moment. This is in plants, the other in metals: foz plants and hearbes, doe wyther and vanish away in a mo= ment : but metalls wil continue a thoufand yeares and moze. Now how can hearbs pzomife long life, & helpe of continuance, which they themfelues dos want? Contrariwife, foz fo much as

metalls

metalls doe fo long preferue themfelues by their long life, why fhuld they not performe the fame,being taken into mens bodies?

The Phylofophers fay,that gold, of all other metalls is moft temperat,by the temperatures wherof,the balfam which is in vs waxing ficke, that is to fay degenerating from his temperature by the force of ficknefles,is reftored & holpen,in fuch wife,that the vertue of his medicine doth recall him to his temper,and doth fo increafe him with ftrength, that he eafily ouercōmeth ficknefle. Gold is confecrated to the Sunne for his colour and brightnefle, and to *Iupiter* for his temperature,& therefore it can wonderfully temper the natural heate with moyfture, preferue the humours from corruption, and bring the Solary and Iouial vertue to the fpirits and members.

The beft way to make potable gold,is without mixture of any other thing.The next vnto potable gold,is that which is beaten into thin leaues,which for want of the other, may be vfed in medicine cordial,to comfort the heart.The tincture of gold being extracted, doth clenfe and reftore the blood. So that hereby the homogenial and kindly parts are gathered together , and the Heterogenial or vnkindly are feperated.For ther is nothing vnder heauen to be found more homogenial , or fimular, of more thinne fubftance,of more temperate nature,& lefle fubiect to corruption,or putrifaction,then the very pure fubftance of metalls, or quick-filuer. What therefore can be more fit for our Ballam then that fpirituall medicine , purged from all impuritie , and brought to exquifite fubtiltie . Doth not a fpirituall nature reioyce and imbrace a fpirituall nature?Why is not gold impayred in the fier, but doth rather ioy therein, and is made more pure ? Is it not becaufe it is fier ? For fier is not thruft out with fier, but they imbrace one the other as being of one kind. So in like manner,for fo much as our Ballam of life is moft pure,and refembleth the nature of fier,why fhould it not receiue his like, and be ftrengthened thereby? For *Geber* faith,that gold is a medicine,which maketh the heart merry, & preferueth the body in youth:the which medicine is no other thing,but a natural heat,multiplyed in ŷ fixed fubftance of Mercury:the vertue of which heat is to gather together(as it is faidafore)ŷkindly,&to

difceuer

diſſeuer and put away all things that are vnkindly, conſer-
uing the ſpirits and humours in a man ſooner then in the nature
of metalls, becauſe a man by his proper natural heat doth ſeperate the vnkindly ſuperfluities, which metalls by their vnnatu-
ral heat cannot ſeperate.

But let the reader vnderſtand, that our meaning is not to preſcribe this Aurum potabile, for continual foode, but for medicine
onely in time of neede . For it will ſuffice, if it be taken once or
twiſe in the yeare , to prolong our dayes to Neſtorian yeares,
without the yrkeſomneſſe of ſickneſſe.

The Phyloſophers haue not onely called this medicine Aurum potabile, but alſo the water of life, the Tincture, the preti-
ous ſtone, the medicine which worketh wonderfully vpon three
ſorts of things, namely vpon the animal, vegetable, and minerall: for the which cauſe it is called the Animal, Vegetable, and
Mineral Stone : and the Arabian Aſtrologians call it the great
Elixir.

Wonderful is the vertue of this medicine : for herewith the
body of man being ſick, is reſtored to health , imperfect metals
are turned into gold or ſiluer , and vegetables, albeit they are
dry and withered, being moyſtened with this liquor, doe waxe
freſh and græne againe. This Medicine being a quinteſſence is
almoſt incorruptible and immortal , temperate, purified by the
elements themſelues, and ſeperated from the dregs and groſſe
matter of the fower elements, which are the moſt chiefe cauſe of
corruption, as the Phyloſophers affirme : which therefore maketh a temperate and ſound body, becauſe it is, as it were the ſpirit of life, by whoſe force and helpe, nature doth digeſt all that is
indigeſted, or expulſe the ſuperfluous and offending humours: it
ſuppreſſeth their qualities, it quickeneth the ſpirit, it maketh the
ſoft hard, and the hard ſoft: the thick, thinne, and the thinne thick:
the leane fat , and the fat leane: it maketh the cold, hote, and the
hote cold: it moyſteneth the dry, and dryeth the moyſt: to conclude,
it confirmeth and ſtrengtheneth the natural heate & moyſture.
And as all Phyloſopers doe write with one conſent, it is an vniuerſal medicinable body, whereunto all the particularities of medicines, are reduced and infuſed.   For

For this cause,it is as it were a finely nature, or essence, a most thinne soule,most purgatiue, much resisting for a very long time, putrifaction or corruption, freed from al mortal concreti-on, a celestial and simple substance of the Elements, brought to to this spiritual nature,by *(chymical sublimation.*

And yet for al this, we affirme not that this medicine is al-together incorruptible, for as much as it is made and consisteth of natural things. Neuerthelesse, it is brought to that subtiltie, thinnesse and simplicitie spiritual, that it seemeth to containe no-thing in it that is Heterogenial, or vnkindely, whereby it may be corrupted : whereby also it commeth to passe, that being gi-uen to the sicke,it preserueth them a long time in health.

And for this cause the Philosophers haue had this in so great esteeme, and haue wholy addicted themselues to seeke and search out the same, not to make themselues rich, by turning imperfect metals into gold and siluer, when as many of them willingly embraced pouertie, but rather to heale the diseases and sicknes-ses of men, and to defende and preserue their liues in long health without griefe, vnto the time which God hath appointed.

But leauing this great mysterie,which very fewe attaine vn-to, I wil in charitie and good wil deliuer here vnto thee, an easie prescription how to make certaine waters,of great vertue,which I found written in the Latine tongue, in an auncient coppy : seruing to keepe the body in health, and to deliuer it from many infirmities, which I thought good here to insert , as very perti-nent to this Treatise , which concerneth (as you haue heard) the vertue of Minerals.

Take of *Aqua vitæ*, distilled with red Wine,*lib.*4. Of burnt Salt, *lib.*2. Of dead Sulphur,*lib* 2. Of white Tartar. ʒ. 2. Of the coales of Flaxe which groweth in *Abella*, a Towne of *Cam-pania* in *Italie*; ʒ. 3. Of Salt Peter,ʒ.4. Beate al these into fine pouder, & searc them : and being mingled together, powre on them the aforesaid *Aqua vitæ*, and so put the whole masse to distillation.

The Vertues of the Diſtillation.

THe firſt Diſtilation, hath vertue of a *Balſam* to conſerue both fleſh and Fiſh, from putrifaction. It clenſeth the face from all freckles and ſpots, clearing the ſkinne, and making it fairer. It cleanſeth the body from Itch and Scabbes, and dryeth vp the teares, and watrineſſe of the eyes.

The ſecond diſtillation expelleth impoſtumations, and ſuperfluities of the body, faſteneth the teeth which are loſe, and taketh away the windineſſe of the Liuer.

The third taketh away a ſtinking breath, and purgeth tough flegme out of the Stomach, and whatſoeuer is not wel digeſted.

The fourth expelleth blood which is congealed in the body.

The fifth healeth and taketh away from man the faling ſickneſſe.

The ſixt diſtillation helpeth al paines about the throate.

The ſeuenth cureth the paine of the Goute.

The eight is an excellent *Balſam*, which ſee thou keepe well.

The ninth diſtillation comforteth and preſerueth the Liuer, if a little gold be diſſolued therein.

After euery of the former diſtillations, the feces muſt be beaten, and ſearced as in the beginning.

Another Water, by which a Phiſitian may worke wonders.

TAke the filings of Siluer, of Braſſe, of Iron, of Leade, of Steele, of Gold, the ſumme or froth of Golde, and of Siluer, and of Storax: ſo much of all theſe as the abilitie of the man can wel affoorde: put theſe the firſt day in the vrine of ſeuen yeares of age: the ſecond day, in white Wine, made hote: the third day, into the Iuice of Fennel: the fourth day, into the white of an Egge: the fifth day, into womans milke which giueth a boy ſucke: the ſixth day, into red wine: the ſeuenth day, in ſeuen whites of Egges. Then put all this into a cupel, and diſtill diſtil it with a ſoft and gentle fyer. That which is diſtilled keepe in a Siluer oꝛ golden veſſel. There cannot bee ſpoken enough in the pꝛaiſe of this water. It cureth all ſoꝛtes of Lepꝛoſie, and wonderfully clenſeth the body. It maketh youth to continue long. Uſe it to thy comfoꝛt, and to the good of thy neighbour.

CHAP. XVIII.

Shewing by what remedies ſickneſſes are to be cured.

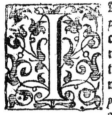 IT is alleaged out of the authoꝛitie of *Hypocrates* and *Galen*, that contraries are cured by contraries. But hee which affirmeth that contraries are cured by contraries, hee ſhall neuer eaſily finde out a remedie foꝛ ſickneſſe: neither was this *Hypocrates* meaning, as ſhall bee ſhewed anon. It is out of queſtion that ſickneſſes doe ariſe from the diſagrement of the beginnings: and ſo often as thoſe beginnings doe decline from their temper, (which is then called a diſtemperature) and the one being ſeperated from the conſoꝛt of the other, taking vp his ſtanding by himſelfe, pꝛocureth ſickneſſe. Foꝛ when it is not in mixture with the other, (which being ioyned together, do maintaine concoꝛd) they then make warre vpon the body, without any ſtoppe oꝛ let. I ſpeake not here of ſimple and bare qualities, but of the very eſſences wherein are thoſe powers and faculties whereof *Hypocrates* ſpeaketh, which pꝛeſerue the health of their *Balſam*, oꝛ to reſtoꝛe it when it is loſt.

Seeing therefoꝛe the ſedes and pꝛoperties both of health and of ſickneſſes, lye hid in the eſſences, it followeth that they are to be cheriſhed in eſſences, and not with qualities. The which eſſences foꝛſomuch as they are meere acting ſpirits, they are to be repelled

with

with ſpirits, not with bodyes, which are not like them, oz which are contrary to them.

But it is obiected, that al things conſiſt of Elements, therefoze our bodies alſo. If then the Element of ayer do ſuffer and be out of courſe in vs, ſhal the ſame be holpen with the Element of earth? Why then haue Phiſitians ſo fewe remedies againſt the peſtilence? Is it becauſe there are none at al? (I confeſſe when God wil puniſh hee taketh away the vertue from remedies and medicines.) That is not the cauſe, I meane the want of remedies, but becauſe ignozant Phiſitians, know not the cauſes of the peſtilence, and therefoze dee not rightly pzouide to pzeuent the ſame. Foz ſeeing they oppoſe againſt the peſtilence comming of the cozruption of the Ayer, a medicine taken from earth, water oz ayer, oz from the earth hauing a watery oziginal, what maruayle is it, if there follow no effect thereof, when as they doe not dziue away thoſe things which are to bee mixed together, but thoſe things which dee eaſily agree and are gathered together. Foz how can the heauen and the earth bee mingled together, to helpe the diſtemperature of the Heauen, betwéene the which there is ſo great diſtance, as there is betwéen diuiſible and indiuiſible, as *Plato* ſpake. Therefoze celeſtiall things are to be mingled with celeſtial things, waterie with waterie, and earthie with earthie, and not contrariwiſe, otherwiſe there can be no agréement.

Conſider wel, that Heauen, Aier, Water, and Earth, are in vs, but yet a certaine thing alſo farre moze excellent, namely, a certaine ſupernatual body, which conſerueth all other things in their temperature, whoſe ſtrength retaineth a'l other things in their office: whereas imbecilitie and defect ſuffereth them to be out of courſe. What then is to bee done in this conflict but to cheriſh and vphold in his vigoz and ſtrength, that ſupernatural bodie, that is to ſay, the *Balſam* of nature, that al other things ſubiect thereunto, and to whom it giueth life, may by the meane thereof be continued in their eſtate, firme and ſound? But with what things ſhall the imbecilitie and defect thereof be reſtozed, but with things of the ſame likeneſſe?

All

Doth Oyle increase by putting water therein ? Doth not one enemie put another to flight, euen as one friend helpeth another? Al sicknesses come hereof in our bodie, in what soeuer they be seated, because the *Balsam* of nature and life, doe there decay and decrease. What else then is to be done, but to helpe our weake friend?

Hypocrates sayth, that hunger is a sicknesse. For whatsoeuer doth put a man to paine, deserueth the name of sicknesse: whatsoeuer then aswageth hunger, is a remedie for this sicknesse, such is al maner of food, wherewith that sicknesse is cured. ⟨*Lib. de flat. bus.*⟩

Therefore according to the opinion of *Hypocrates*, foode is a remedie. But wherefore are meates and drinkes sayde to bee medicinal remedies, but because they haue natural properties, agréeing with the *Balsam* of nature, not contrarie, wherby the weakened forces and strength are corroborated and the defect thereof restored. After the same manner drinke alayeth thirst. Why and how commeth this to passe but onely hereof, because as nourishment is all one with that which is nourished, so thirst is al one with the humour wanting, or with drinke?

Hereby wée sée how wrong their iudgement is, which apply contraries to contraries, to strengthen nature, that it may frée it selfe from sicknesse. Which nature if shée should séeke helpe for an enemie, she must néedes fall into a greater perrill, than if she were to try the combate onely with sicknesse. And yet for all this wée reiect not the saying of *Hypocrates*, that contraryes, must haue contrarie remedies: that is to say, by the taking away of the diseasefull impurities, and by the repairing of the strength and natural *Balsam*, not by calefaction, or refrigeration, by humectation, or exsiccation: not by abstersion, incision, attenuation, by such other like, too common & familiar to *Galen*.

But we are of *Hypocrates* minde, that hunger is cured by meate, thirst with drinke, repletion with euacuation, emptines with refection, labour with rest, and rest with labour. The which ⟨*Hip. lib. de Antiq med. dicina.*⟩ of some are not vnderstood, as they are expounded of *Galen*, who applyeth those contrarieties to those bare qualities whereof *Hypocrates* speaketh, séeing a medicine is nothing else, then an ap-

D   position

poſition of thoſe things which are deſired, & an ablation of thoſe things which doe too much abound, accoʒding to the ſound opinion of *Galen* here.

But *Hypocrates* aymeth at a further matter, in that he wou'd haue the diſeaſe qualified & dʒiuen away, by giuing ſtrength to nature againſt the enemy: which nature being the onely Phyſitian and curer of diſeaſes, is to be holpen with ſuch things as are like to the diſeaſes, that ſo ſickneſſes and the paſſions of ſickneſſes may be mittigated: euen as hunger and thʒſt, are recreated & aſſwaged by thoſe remedies, which they grædily deſire. But hoſtile things, that are enemy & contrary, are not deſired, but ſuch things as are a friend and familiar. Foʒ who wil giue to his hungery ſon when he aſketh bʒead, a *Scorpion?* Therefoʒe. like and fitting liquoʒs, and nouriſhments are to be giuen, which may pʒocure to nature deſired reſt. Foʒ remedies which come out of the ſame fountaine, and out of the ſame familie, which are agræing and fitting in likeneſſe are to be miniſtred. Foʒ the thʒſting ſpirits of feuers, are to be recreated with ſyʒups, with ſugars, with pertiſan alone, oʒ with wine, becauſe they are not of the ſame family and affinitie with them, therefoʒe neither familiar friends noʒ kinſmen: but with thoſe tart liquoʒs, which are begotten of the ſame linage, which are ſpiritual not coʒpoʒal, as are thoſe foʒmer, of the which, if certaine dʒops be offered to him which is a thirſt, they wil by and by ſlake his thirſt, and pʒeſently bʒing ſuch thirſty ſpirits to their reſt. After the ſame maner, watchings, paines, burning heates, and ſuch like are cured. Foʒ when the ſpirits are thirſty, that is to ſay, when they deſire any thing like to themſelues which is wanting, they wil neuer be appeaſed noʒ at reſt, vntill they haue obtained that which they deſire, and haue ſupplyed their want. Wherefoʒe they are rightly called, by *Hypocrates*, contraries: and by *Hermeticall* Phyſitians, remedies of like ſoʒt. Foʒ they are Similies, which are dʒawen from the ſame anatomie of nature, contayning like pʒoperties, tinctures, and rootes. And on the other ſide, they are contraries, becauſe they ſupply the defects, and doe ſatiſfie the deſires with friendly fulneſſe, appeaſing the ſpirits, and their fitting

impurities,

impurities, ſæking to conſume them, oꝛ to take them away.
Wherefoꝛe theſe phꝛaſes of ſpæch in natures anatomie, albeit
they ſæme different, and repugnant one to the other, yet in god
conſent and agræement they are receiued and admitted. That is
to ſay, that contraries haue contrary remedies, ꝛ like to their like.

But to returne to our beginning, that is to ſay to the elements,
oꝛ to thoſe thꝛæ hypoſtatical ꝑ foꝛmal pꝛinciples of bodies, namely Salt, Sulphur, and Mercurie, which is a liquoꝛ: foꝛ ſo much as
vpon them all grieuous diſeaſes foꝛ the moſt part doe depend, in
ſo much that a comon peſtilence flying in the outward aire cannot inuade a man, but it muſt make a bꝛeach and aſſaile one of
theſe. Therefoꝛe thou ſhalt not doe moꝛe fooliſhly, if to helpe him
which is grieued with a mercurial ſickneſſe, thou vſe a remedie
taken out of Sulphur, then if thou ſhouldeſt mingle oyle with
water, which two wil neuer be mixed oꝛ vnited. And in like ſoꝛt,
thou ſhalt labour in vaine, if thou goe about to helpe Sulphurus
ſickneſſes with a Mercurial medicine: oꝛ to put away ſalt ſickneſſes with the help of others. Foꝛ theſe wil neuer agræ together: and being ſo valike one to the other, they wil neuer be ioyned in one, to heale and cure the bodie, except they be knit in a
friendly peace and vnion, by that ſupernatural ꝑ ethereal body,
that is to ſay, by the *Balſam* which is common to al things. Hæ
therefoꝛe which is ſick of Mercurie, muſt be holpen with mercurial remedies: as the *Epilepſie*, and the *Apolexi*, are to be holpen
with vitriolated remedies taken from water. And hæ which
wil help ſulphurus ſickneſſe, muſt vſe ſulphurus remedies, and
ſickneſſes pꝛocæding of Salt, with medecines taken from Salt.
So thou ſhalt be taught by reaſon and experience, that things of
like ſoꝛt wil agræ, ꝑ be cured with their like. We might yet make
theſe things moꝛe plaine, ꝑ lay the ſame moꝛe open by many reaſons and examples: but why ſhould we eaſe you of that labour
which we haue vndergon our ſelues by diligẽt reading, ſearching
and experimenting the things of nature, with great expences, befoꝛe we attained our deſire. Accept my god wil in this, which
I frœly offer foꝛ ſome eaſe of thy paines, and foꝛ thy pꝛofit.
And if it fit not thy humour ꝑ taſte (foꝛ al men haue not
one reliſh) leaue it foꝛ thoſe which ſhall
better allow it.

FINIS.   D. 2.

THE SECOND
part of this Treatiſe,
wherein is contained in ſome meaſure the praĉtiſe of the Hermeticall Phyſicke.

CHAP. I.

Alt (whereof hath bene ſpoken before at
large) is a thing of ſuch qualitie, and ſo ex-
cellent in it ſelfe, that all creatures by a certaine natural inſtinĉt, doe deſire the ſame as
a Balſam, by which they are preſerued, conſerued, & doe grow and increaſe. They loue
it, and like it ſo wel (I ſay) that they long af-
ter it, and doe drawe it vnto them by their breath, and doe licke
it with their tongue out of walles, and old rubbiſh. Byrdes, as
Doues and ſuchlike, doe ſearch after it with their beakes, and
wil (if they can) attaine it, though out of feculent places, which
are made fat by mens excrements and vertues. What huge
multitudes of fiſhes are bread and nouriſhed in the Salt Sea?
The which being ſo apparant, I wonder that men are of ſo per-
uerſe iudgement, that they knowe not, or at leaſt will not acknowledge, the admirable effeĉts, of this radical balſam of nature. And who wil not admire the vertual properties and qualities of Salt, yea euen of that which is extraĉted out of liuing creatures: which qualities are to be ſeene in making liquide, in clen-

D 3   ſing

I
Salt hath life in it & is animal.

ſing, in binding, in cutting, in pearcing, in pꝛeſeruing from all coꝛruption, and in attracting, purging, and euacuating? Are not all theſe faculties and many others ſufficient, to pꝛoue that Salt is a thing animal? And ſo much the rather, becauſe there haue bene ſome chiefe Phyloſophers, who haue affirmed the Magnes oꝛ Loadſtone to be animate, oꝛ indued with life, onely becauſe it hath power to dꝛaw pꝛon to it. How many faculties far greater then theſe, yea and the ſame magnetical alſo, do we find in Salt, if we looke diligently and thꝛoughly into them? What is greater, and moꝛe admirable then the Salt of mans bꝛine? which after conuenient pꝛeparation, is made fit to diſſolue gold and ſiluer? which by this their ſimpathy and concoꝛdance, do ſufficiently declare, and manifeſtly giue attraction, and magnetical vertue, occaſioned oꝛ cauſed by their coniunction and copulation. Who ſeeth not thoſe admirable things, which are to be diſcerned, and which fal out in the pꝛeparation thereof, and in the exaltation, whether you reſpect ſo great variety of colours, oꝛ the coagulations, and diſſolutions, when the ſpirit returneth into the body, and the body paſſeth againe into ſpirit: *Chriſtophorus Pariſienſis*, that great Phyloſopher, did not in vaine take the ſubiect here-hence, and begin the foundation of his woꝛke. Thus I hope I haue ſufficiently declared, that our Salt may be ſaide to be animate.

2
Salt is alſo vegetal.

Salt the original matter of pearles and corail.

But that it may appeare alſo to be as vegetal, as it is animal; that is to ſay, that it is not depꝛiued of the growing facultie, it may hereby be demonſtrated, becauſe it is the firſt mouing thing in nature, which maketh to grow, and ſo multiply, and therefoꝛe ſerueth foꝛ the generation of all things: ſo as with the Poets and auncient Phyloſophers it may be ſaid, that *Venus* the mother, and firſt beginner of al generation, is begotten of the Salt ſpume oꝛ froath of the male, the which alſo *Atheneus* confirmeth. Foꝛ this cauſe *Venus* was called by the *Greekes Aligene*, as affianced to the Salt ſea. And alſo the generation of moſt pꝛecious pearles in the ſhels of fiſhes, and of coꝛal ſpꝛinging out of the bowels of hard ſtones and rockes in the ſea, ſpꝛeading foꝛth bꝛanches like a tree.

Hermeticall phyſicke.

trée, doe yet moze and moze confirme this ſentence. Theſe are
the effects, which that fier of nature, Salt, bzingeth forth, yea
euen in the middeſt of moſt cold water.

But let vs ſée alſo what it wozketh in the earth. The effects
which it hath in the earth are theſe : namely, it heateth and maketh the earth fat: it animateth, foztifieth, and giueth power vnto
it : It increaſeth and giueth a vegetating and growing vertue
with ſéede into euery thing in the ſame. Foz what other thing is
it which maketh the earth fatte, and bzingeth to paſſe, that one
graine multiplyeth into a hundzed, but a certaine ſtercozation,
and ſpzeading of dung and of bzine which commeth from cattle?
What other thing openeth the earth and maketh it to ſpzoute in
the beginning of the ſpzing time, after that the Sunne is exalted
into the ſigne of *Aries* (which ſigne is the fall of *Saturn*, and the
houſe of *Mars*, ſignes altogether fiery) but the eleuations and
ſublimations of the ſpirits of the ſaid Salt, and of the balſam of
nature? This is that which giueth heate and quickeneth, which
maketh to grow, and which decketh and ioyeth the medowes
and the fieldes, and which pzoduceth that moſt ample and vniuerſal vigoz and vertue.

Who ſeeth not this in the very aier alſo, by the ſublimations
of the ſpirits of the ſame nature of Salt, which ſpirits being ſu-
blenated into aier in the ſaid ſpzing time, doe fal againe in fozme
of a deawe, vpon cozne and all things that ſpzing out of the earth?
And who ſeeth not that theſe deawes aryſing from the earth,
and falling againe from the aier, is a cauſe of vegetation and
growing? But that the dewe is the ſpirit of the fozeſaid Salt, and
indued with Salt, they which thinke themſelues great Philoſophers, againſt their wils and not without ſhame, do confeſſe,
when they ſée that the true Phyloſophers doe extract out of the
deawe a Salt, which diſſolueth cozall and pearles, no leſſe then
doth the Salt which is extracted out of common Salt, out of
Salt-Péter, out of Miter, oz out of other Salts which are pzepared foz the ſame end.

Furthermoze, the ſame Salt, may rightly alſo be ſaid to bee
vegetall,

Salt the fier of nature.

The effects of Salt in the earth.

The effects of Salt in the aier.

vegetall,becauſe it is manifeſtly found in all vegetables: and becauſe thoſe things in the which it doth moſt abound, haue the
longer life and continuance,and doe moꝛe manifeſtly ſhew foꝛth
the vegetable effects, either in their owne pꝛoper nature, oꝛ at
ſuch times as they are to ſerue foꝛ vſe.

3
Salts mine-
rall.

Salt alſo is well known to be metallick oꝛ minerall. And all
men knowe it the better ſo to be, foꝛ that ſuch ſundꝛy and diuers kinds of Salts are found in the bowels of the earth: ſuch
are Salt, Gem,Allum,Witriol, Salt niter,and ſuch others moe,

Salts of di-
uers kinds.

all which are of metallick nature, oꝛ elſe doe participate much
with the ſame. But a Phyloſopher knoweth how to ranſacke
this thing further, and to find out the innermoſt ſecret hereof by
the helpe of diuers ſtrong waters, which hee knoweth how to
pꝛepare: which are nothing elſe, but the ſpirits of the foꝛeſaids
Salts which haue power to diſſolue and to bꝛing metallick bo-

Stirring wa-
ters.

dies into waters, as is knowns to euery one.I ſay,that by this
diſſolution, we may behold the concoꝛdance & ſimpathy of theſe
Salts,with the metallick nature.Foꝛ becauſe they are like,they
wil be wel mingled together, conioyned and vnited, diſſoluing
his like, and aſſociating himſelfe to his like. Foꝛ ſtrong waters
doe neuer woꝛke vpon wood, oꝛ vpon any other matter, which
is not of metallick nature:As it was moſt truly ſaid of a certaine

Nature ac-
cordeth with
nature.

great Phyloſopher,Nature loueth her like,and delighteth in her
owne nature, And by another wittily thus ſpoken: Eaſie is the
paſſage of things one into the other, which are one in likeneſſe.
Sulphur,and other things, which are of an oyle-like nature,are
ſooner and better diſſolued with oyles, as with the oyles of Te-
rebinth and of Flaxe,oꝛ Linſede,which is moſt ſwéete, then with
that great foꝛce, and moſt violent ſharpneſſe of ſtrong waters,
which are nothing elſe but the ſpirits of Salts, and by conſe-
quent doe diſagrée with Sulphur, which is a beginning contrary to the ſaid ſpirits. Here is offered large occaſion of diſpute,if
time and place would ſerue,but I omit it.

Salt is fuſible

Let vs returne to our Salt: the which if I ſhal ſhew that it
may be moulten and diſſolued,no leſſe then gold and ſiluer, with
the foꝛce of fire, and being cold againe, may be congealed into a
maſſe,

maſſe, as metalls be, then no doubt it wil euidently appeare; that Salt is of a metallick nature. And this I ſay is to be done, not onely in Salt which is found in mines and in caues of the earth, but alſo in the very Salt of the Sea. But for ſo much as the ſame is better knowne to them that haue but meane ſkil in metalls, then that I ſhal neede at this time to ſpend much labour about it, I ceaſe to ſpeake any word more thereof.

Hereby it doth appeare very euidently, that this opinion of *Ariſtotle* is falſe, where he ſaith, that cold diſſolueth the things which are congealed with heate : and that thoſe things which are coagulated by cold, are diſſolued by heate. The which notwithſtanding we grant to be true on the one part, for that wee knowe well, that Salt which is coagulated or congealed by the heate of the Sunne, is diſſolued in cold water. But it muſt bee confeſſed alſo to be true, that Salt, by the vehemencie of the heat of fier, is to be diſſolued, moulten and made flexible, and to be caſt into a moulten lumpe, as eaſily as metalls be.

Moreouer Salts may be extracted out of all calcined metals which are to be diſſolued, filtred, and coagulated, after the ſame manner as are other ſalts, whether they be common and not moulten, or whether they be moulten by the force of heate. For it is knowne to a *Chymiſt* of ſmal practiſe, that out of one pound of calcined lead, tenne or twelue ounces of Salt may be extracted. All which things doe ſufficiently demonſtrate and proue, that the nature of Salt is metallick: and that therefore metall is nothing elſe but a certaine fuſil Salt. Salts may be extracted out of metalls

By that which hath bene ſpoken, it may eaſily appeare, how Salt is animal, vegetal, and mineral, and that it agreeth with that which all the Phyloſophers haue decreed with one conſent concerning the matter and ſubiect of the vniuerſal Medicine.

And hereunto tend all other ſignes, whereby they deſcribe their foreſaid matter, albeit moſt obſcurely. All which things to agree with the nature of Salt: as that it is of ſmal eſtimation: that it is to be found in euery thing, and in our ſelues: the which is moſt plaine, for ſo much as there is nothing compounded in

this

vniuerſal woʒld, out of the which, and at all times, Salt cannot be extracted.

CHAP. II.

The three principles of all things are contained
in Salt, extracted out of the
earth.

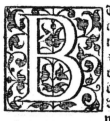

Ut to ſhewe now moʒe particularly thoſe things whereof we haue ſpoken generally, namely, that Salt doe participate with the animal, vegetal, and mineral nature, wee wil vſe a common example, the which notwithſtanding, being exactly and diligently waighed and conſidered by a true Phyloſopher, is a notable miſtery. The which, albeit it bee taken from out of the earth, yet it may lift vp our eyes to heauen.

I meane to ſpeake of Niter, which men commonly cal Salt Pæter. I let paſſe the deteſtable and pernicious vſe thereof, inuented foʒ the deſtruction of men: And yet I muſt confeſſe that it deſerueth great admiration, in that it ſheweth foʒth ſo great, and incredible effects. when as we being in theſe lower parts, it repreſenteth thʒanoʒings and lightenings, as if they were in the aire aloft. But if we ſhould conſider what it is, and of what quality, in his owne nature and compoſition, what diuers facu'ties, and qualities, and effects there are in a thing ſo vile and ſo common, it would no doubt make vs to wonder out of meaſure.

Niter is made and compounded of earth his mother, which bʒingeth foʒth the ſame: oʒ it is taken out of old rubbiſh grounds, oʒ out of places where ſtables foʒ beaſts haue bene, oʒ out of ſuch

kind

kind of groundes which haue bene replenished with salt liquor, or with the brine of beastes, rather then out of a leane hungry land, washed with raine, or by some such like occasion, deprived of that radicall humour. It is most plentifully extracted from the ground where doue-houses are seated, and out of Pigeons dung: and this is the best Piter of all others : the which is worthy the noting. Whereby it appeareth, that Piter doth participate with the excrements and brines of liuing creatures.

For brines are nothing else , but a superfluous seperation of the Salt of vegetables , by which, liuing creatures are nourished and doe liue . Whereby it euidently appeare, how the foresaid Salt doth in kind participate with the nature animal, and vegetable . For as touching that which pertaineth to the mineral, it is not much pertinent to our purpose to speake thereof, sauing that wee thinke good to adde thus much , that it is extracted out of the earth, which is the reason why it is called Salt-Péeter, when as more properly it should be called the salt of the earth. But let vs goe forward.

Nature ministereth matter to Art, whereof Salt-Péeter is compounded : Art cannot make by it selfe, no more then nature can make Salt-Péeter-pure, and seperated from all terrestrilie and heterogeneal or vnkindly substance . For that it may produce the same effects which the other produceth, it must be prepared by the industry of workemen . For these make choyse of conuenient earth, and out of fit places, to them well knowne , and being filtered, or strained with hote common water, againe and againe, through the same earth , as lyes are vsually made with ashes , it commeth to passe that a saltnesse or brinish taste is mingled therewith, which is proper to all salts.

Of the which like, or water so distreined, if two thirds or thereaboutes be vapored away by seething at the fire , and then let coole, the salt will be thickened into an Ice, whereof the maker of Salt-Péeter finisheth his worke, purifying the same by sundry dissolutions, and coagulations, that it may loose his fatnesse quite and cleane.

This

This common worke, being triuial, and no better then mechanical, if it be rightly considered and weighed, is (as I haue said already) full of admiration. For by the very same preparation, the three beginnings are extracted out of earth, which may be seperated one from the other, and yet neuerthelesse the whole three, doe consist in one and the same essence, and are onely distinguished in properties and vertues. And herein we may plainly see as in a glasse (after a certaine manner) that in comprehensible misery of the three persons in one and the same Hypostasis or substance, which make the diuine Trinitie. For thus it hath pleased the omnipotent Creator, to manifest and shewe himselfe a vnitrine, or Triune, not onely herein, that he is found so to be in the nature of earth, but vniuersally in all the workes of the creation. For this our comparison of the Salt of the earth is general, and is euery where found, and in all things.

A Figure of the Trinitie.

Also in this comparison of Salt, wee may beholde three distinct natures, which neuerthelesse are and doe subsist in one and the same essence. For the first nature is Salt common, fixed, and constant: and the other nature is Volatil Salt, the which alone, the Sal-peeter-man seeketh after.

Three distinct natures in Salt.

This volatil or flying Salt, containeth in it two kindes of Volatil Salt: the other full of Sulphur, easily catching flame, which men call Niter: the other Mercurial, watery, sower partaking of the nature of Salt Armoniac.

Wherefore in that most common essence of earth, these three seueral Salts are found, vnder one and the same nature of the which three, all vegetables and animalls whatsoeuer doe participate. And we determine to place our three hypostatical and substantial beginnings, vpon these three Salts, as vpon the fundamental grounds, in that our worke, concerning the hidden nature of things, and the misteries of Art, the which we had thought to haue published before this time: whereof we thought it conuenient to say some thing by the way, because the groundworke and beginnings of Medicines depend vpon them.

Where-

Hermeticall Physicke.

Wherefore to the end so large & immeasurable doctrine, may the better and more diligently be considered of all men, especially of the wiser sort, then heretofore it hath bene, I wil set plainly before their eyes, those three distinct natures of Salt, comprehended (as already is sayd) in one *Hypostasis*, or substance.

For the maker of Salt-peter, or Niter, to make his salt the more effectual, volatile, and more apt to take fire, taketh away the saltnesse (as they terme it) from the same, and separateth the Salt thereof, which is al one with the sea salt, or common salt, which is dissolued into common water: Contrariwise, Salt-peter (as men cal it) is congealed into such peeces, as we see it to be: and so there is made a visible seperation of both the Salts. For the water (wherein the common Salt being defused and dissolued as we said) being euaporated or boyled away, there remayneth a portion of Salt in the bottome, which is somewhat like to our common marine Salt, and of the nature thereof, for it hath the same brynish qualities, it is fixed, it melteth not in the fire, *Two salts appeare in the making of salt peter.* neither is it set on fire, and therefore is wholy different from that which is congealed in the same water, which is called Salt-peter. The which thing truly deserueth to bee diligently considered, not of ordinary Salt-peter-men, which are ignorant of the nature of things, but of Philosophers, if they desire to be reputed, and to be such. To whom it shal manifestly appeare, that Salt which by nature and qualitie (according to the common opinion of Philosophers) is hote and dry, a sulphurus Salt, fierie, and apt to be set on fire, such as is Salt peter, wil be coagulated or congealed in water, wherein al other saltes are dissolued, no lesse than that salt which proceded from the very same essence of Salt-peter, may be dissolued in water, as we haue said.

Therefore not without great cause, the admirable nature of Salt-peter deserueth to be considered, which comprehendeth in it two volatile partes: the one of Sulphur, the other of Mercurie. The Sulphurus part is the soule thereof, the Mercurial is his spirit. *Two flying parts of salt-peter.*

The Sulphurus part commeth to that first mouing of nature, which is nothing else, but an ethereal fire, which is neither

P 3. hote

Sulphur of Nature.

hote no2 d2ie, not conſuming like the Elementarie fy2e, but is a certaine Celeſtial fy2e, and Ayerie humour, hote and moyſte, and ſuch as wée may almoſt beholde in *Aqua Vitæ*; a fy2e, I ſay, contempered, ful of life, which in Uegetables, wée cal the begetating ſoule: in Animals, the hote and moyſt radical: the natural and unnatural heate, the true Nectar of life, which falling into any ſubiect, whether it bée Animal o2 Uegetable, death by and by enſueth. The which commeth ſo to paſſe uppon no other cauſe, but uppon the defect of this vital heate, which is the repay2er and conſeruer of life.

The Mercurial part of ſalt-peter.

The ſame vital heate, is alſo to bée found, albeit mo2e obſcurely in Minerals: which may mo2e eaſily bée comp2ehended by the ſympathy and conco2dance, which the layd ſalt-peter hath with Mettals: as is to be ſéene in the diſſolutions, whereof wée haue ſpoken ſomewhat befo2e.

Beſide that ſulphurus part, there is alſo found in ſalt-peter, a certaine Mercurial o2 ayerie nature, and which notwithſtanding cannot take fy2e, but is rather contrary thereunto. This ſpirit is not hote in qualitie, but rather colde, as appeareth by the tart and ſharpe taſte thereof: the which ſharpneſſe and coldneſſe is wonderful, and is farre different from the Elementary coldneſſe: fo2 that it can diſſolue bodies, and coagulate ſpirites, no leſſe then it doth congeale ſalt-peter: the which ſowerneſſe is the generall cauſe of *Fermentation*, and coagulation of al natural things.

The cauſe of ferment, is ſowerneſſe.

This ſame ſower and tart ſpirit, is alſo found in ſulphurs, of the ſame qualitie, not burning, no2 ſetting on fire, and which congealeth ſulpur, and maketh it firme, which otherwiſe would bée running like Oyle. Uitriol, among al the kindes of ſalt, doth moſt of al abound with this ſpirit, becauſe it is of the nature of *Venus*, o2 *Copper*: which ſower ſpirit inconſtant *Mercurie* (which notwithſtanding alwayes tendeth to his perfection, that is to ſay, to his coagulation and fixation) ful wel can make choyſe of, and attract it to him, that hée may bée fixed

Vitriol is of the nature of Copper.

fixed and coagulated , when it is mixed and sublimed with the same vitriol . Euen as Bees suck hony from flowers, as *Ripley* saith.

The spirit of Vitriol fixeth Mercurie.

Furthermore, this sharpe, sower, and cold spirit, is the cause why Salt-Peeter hauing his sulphur set on fire, giueth a cracke: that so salt-peeter may be of the number of them , whereof *Aristotle* writeth , as that they are moued with a contrary motion: Which words of his are diligently to be considered . But what doe I meane to open the gate of passage into the orchard of the *Hesperides*, in speaking so plainly of salt-peeter, giuing thereby a free accesse vnto the doltish and ignorant ? Be not therefore deceiued, in taking my words according to the letter. Salt-Peeter of the Phylosophers or fusile salt (whereof at the first came the name of *Halchymie*) is not Salt-Peeter, or that common Niter: yet neuerthelesse, the composition and wonderful nature thereof, is as it were a certaine example, and *Lesbian* rule of our worke. Howbeit I haue spoken more plainly & manifestly vnto you of this matter , then any other which hath gone before me hath done.

Let therefore *Momus* from henceforth hold his peace , and let slaunderous tongues bee hereafter silenced . Also let the ignorant open their eares and eyes, and giue good heede to that which followeth, wherein shal bee plainly shewed many admirable things, and secrets of exceeding great profite. Wherewith bee you wel satisfied, and take my good will in good part, till hereafter I shal deliuer that which shal better content you.

C A H P.

CHAP. III.

Wherein by Examples, the forces and properties
of Salt are manifested.

We haue seene out of that first remaining *Chaos* (that is to say, out of that base earth, or out of a matter confused and deformed) an extraction, and seperation of a fairer, bright cleere, and transparent forme: that is to say, of that Salt, which is apt to receiue many other formes, and which is endued with diuers and wonderfull properties.

Ye haue also seene, how out of one, and the same essence, three distinct and seuerall things, yea, three beginnings of Nature are extracted: of the which all bodyes are compounded, and with skilfull *Chymist* can extract and seperate out of euery naturall bodie, that is to say, out of Mineral, Uegetal, and Animal : to wit, Salt, Sulphur, and Mercurie : principles verily most pure, most simple, and truely Elementarie of Nature, all comprehended vnder one essence of Salt, Sulphur, and Mercurie, which Philosophers are wont to compare with the body, Spirit, and Soule : for the body is attributed to salt : the spirit to Mercurie : and the soule to sulphur : euery one to their apt and conuenient attribute.

Body, soule, and spirit.

And the spirit is as it were the mediator, and conseruer of the soule with the body, because through the benefite thereof, it is ioyned and coupled with the soule. And the soule, quickeneth the spirit, and the body.

We haue also seene in the aforesaide salt, a *Hermaphroditicall* Nature : Male and female : fixed and volatil : Agent and Pacient : and which is more, hot and cold : fier and Ice, by mutual friendship and sumpathie ioyned in one, and vnited into one substance : wherein is to be seene the wonderful nature thereof.

The properties thereof are no lesse wonderfull : nay, rather
much

much moꝛe wonderful. Foꝛ Salt peter is the eſpecial key and cheife Poꝛter, which openeth moſt hard bodies, and the moſt ſolid things, as wel ſtones as Metal: and bꝛingeth gold and ſiluer into liquoꝛ, which the pꝛoper water extracted out of the whole maſſe without ſeparation of the male oꝛ fixed. And as it maketh al boodyes metallick, ſpiritual and volatile: ſo on the contrary part, it hath vertue to fixe and to incoꝛpoꝛate ſpirits, how flying ſoeuer they bee.

Who now wil not wonder, oꝛ rather bee amaꝛed, which knoweth that Salt-peter is ſo apt & reaoy to take fire, by which it paſſeth into ayꝛe and ſmoake, and yet in the meane time ſeeth that it remaineth liquid and ſuſible in a red hote crucible, placed in the center of burning coales¬ notwithſtanding the which moſt burning heate, it conceiueth no flame, except the flame oꝛ fyꝛe happen to touch it. And which is moꝛe, being of nature ſo volati', it is at the length fired, neither is it ouercome by the fire, neither doth it yæloe bee it neuer ſo violent and burning, no moꝛe then doth the *Salamander* (if it be true which is repoꝛted of that beaſt) which befoꝛe notwithſtanding it could not abide, noꝛ by any manner of meanes indure. Thus therefoꝛe yæ ſæ, that by fire onely his nature is transfoꝛmed.

Furthermoꝛe the ſame Salt peter, which was of late rightly pꝛepared and clenſed, ſo white and Chꝛiſtalline, (at the leaſt outwardly ſo appearing) being now put into a ſtꝛatoꝛie fire you ſhal ſæ that it conteineth within it al maner of colours, as græne, red yellow, and white, with many others moe. The which if any man wil hardly beléeue becauſe he wil bæ rather incredulous than docile, I wiſh him to make tryal thereof, and then hæ ſhal learne ſo notable a myſterie of Naʼure, within the ſpace of tenne houres, with very little coſt.

And leaſt yæ ſhould take mæ foꝛ ſome *Lycophrone*, oꝛ *Gramarian* wꝛiter of Tragedies, I wil teach you how ſo woꝛke truely and plainly.

Take of Salt peter the fineſt and cleareſt, one pound oꝛ two; put it into a glaſſe Alembic with a couer, and ſet it in ſand: no otherwiſe than if you ſhould diſtil *Aqua Fortis*. Put fyꝛe vnder, *A practiſe.*

and moderate the same by degrées according to Art: the which
fyre thou shalt increase the third or fourth houre after, in such
wise, til the sand appeare very hote. This fyre in the highest degrée thou shalt continue by the space of fiue or sire houres: and
then thou shalt finde and plainly sée, that the spirits of Salt-peter,
haue penetrated the very glasse of the Alembic, and that it hath
discoloured the same as wel within as without.

Furthermore the spirits of the Salt peter, which are come
through the body of glasse, cleauing to the out side therof like vnto
flower, yée make take off with a soft feather, and easilie gather together in great quantitie. This flower is nothing else, but the spirit of Salt-peter, wherein ye shal sée al sorts of colours very liuely expressed.

That which remaineth in the bottom of the Culcurbit, so white
as snow, and wholy fired, is a special remedie to extinguish al
Feauers. It is giuen from halfe a drachme to a drachme, dissolued in some conuenient liquor.

And to speake in a word, this remedy hath not his like, to cut,
to clense, and to purge, and euacuate the corruptions of humors,
and to conserue the body from al pollution of corruption. For
séeing it is of the nature of Balsamic Salt, it must néedes bée indued with such vertues and properties. And in very déede to
deale plainly and truely, I cannot if I would, sufficiently extol
with prayses, the true Salt-peter, and Fusile salt of the Phylosophers. This Salt, *Homer* cals diuine. And *Plato* writeth,
that this Salt, is a friend and familar to diuine things. And many Phylosophers haue said, that it is the soule of the vniuersal,
the quickening spirit, and that which generateth al things.

It may peraduenture séeme that we haue bene too tedious in
the inquisition and speculation, as wel of the general, as of the
particular, concerning the nature of Salt: but it is so profitable
and necessarie, that it is the Basis, and foundation of al medicinable faculties (as more at large shalbe shewed in his place) that
Physitians may haue wherewith to busie themselues, and to vnderstand.

But as touching a Chymical Philosopher, let him know
that

A good pur-
gation of bad
humours.

that hæ ought to beſtowe his labour moſt chiefely in ſuſil Salts, and to remember that Philoſophers haue not without good cauſe euer and anon cryed; Bake it, Bake it, and bake it againe: which is al one, as if they had ſayd, Calcine, calcine, oz bring it to aſhes.

And in very dæde if wæ wil confeſſe the trueth of the matter, al Chymical woꝛkings, as Diſtillations, Calcinations, Reuerberations, Diſſolutions, Filtrations, Coagulations, Decoctions, Fixations, and ſuch other appertaining to this Science, tend to no other ende. then ſo to bring their bodies into duſt oꝛ aſhes, that they may communicate the ſpirits of Saltes and ſulphur which haue made them (placed neuertheleſſe vnder one and the ſame eſſenes) after a certaine imperceptible manner, with their metallick water, and true Mercurie: and that to this ende, that by the infernal vertue and foꝛce of Salt, the Mercurie may bæ conſumed, boyled, and altered from his vile nature, into a moꝛe noble: when as of common Mercurie, it is made by the benefite of the ſpirit of Salt, the Mercurie of the Philoſophers: which Salt it hath attracted out of the aſhes, oꝛ calx vive Metallick.

Euen like as it commeth to paſſe in the lye-waſh which is made of aſhes and water, the which bæing oftentimes melſhed and oꝛawen away, the aſhes leaue al their life and ſtrength, communicating all their Salt to the foꝛeſayd water: the which water, albeit, it alwayes remaineth fluxile and liquid, yet it abydeth not ſimple and pure water, colde, oꝛ of final vertue: but bæing now made lye, it is become hote, and of a dꝛying qualitie, clenſing, and of qualitie wholely actiue, which is altogether the vertue and facultie of an altering medicine.

But it is to bæ conſidered, of what matter this quicke and metallick aſhes are to bæ made. Alſo of what manner of water the lye is to bæ prepared, that thou mayeſt exalt the Salt oꝛ Sulphur of the Philoſophers, that is to ſay, the Balſamick medicine, which is ful of actiue qualities like vnto thunder, bæing reduced into a true liuing calx.

And whereas at the firſt, it was a certaine dead body voyde of life, it ſhal then be made a liuing body indued with ſpirit, and medicinal vertue.

CHAP. IIII.

Gold animated, is the chiefe ſubiect of the
metallic Medicine of the
Philoſophers.

IF ſo great power and foꝛce is the Phyloſophical Sulphur or Nature, that it multiplyeth and increaſeth gold in ſtrength and vertue, being already indued with great perfection, not ſo much foꝛ the equal concurrencie of Sulphur and Quick-ſiluer, as in regard of the perfect combination, adequation, equabilitie of Elements, and

Gold tryumpheth in earth, in aier and in fire.

of the pꝛinciples which make gold. And the ſayd pꝛinciples oꝛ beginnings (to wit, Salt, Sulphur, and Mercurie,) doe ſo oꝛder themſelues, that the one doth not exceed the other : but being as it were equally ballanced and pꝛopoꝛtionated, they make gold to bæ incoꝛruptible : in ſuch wiſe, that neither the earth (being buried therein) can canker, fret and coꝛrupt it, noꝛ the Ayꝛe alter it, noꝛ yet the fire maiſter it, noꝛ diminiſh the leaſt part of it.

The incorruptibilitie of gold, maketh it the beſt Medicine to helpe a corruptible body.

And the reaſon hereof is, foꝛ that (as the Phyloſopher ſaith) *No equal hath any commaund or maiſterie ouer his equal.* Foꝛ becauſe alſo, in euery body equalled and duly pꝛepoꝛtioned, no action oꝛ paſſion can be found; Alſo this is onely that equalitie, which *Pithagoras* called the Mother, the Nurce, and the defender of the concoꝛd of al things. This is the cauſe that in gold and in euery perfect body, wherein this equalitie is, there is a certaine incontrollable and incoꝛruptible compoſition. The which when the ancient Phyloſophers obſerued, they ſought foꝛ that great and incomparable Medicine in gold.

And

And becauſe they vnderſtood, that gold was of ſo ſmal compacted and firme compoſition, that it could not worke, and ſend
his effects into our body, ſo long as it remained in that ſolidity,
they ſought & indeuored to diſſolue and breake his hard bones,
and by the benefit of vegetable Sulphur, and by the artificious
working of the Balſam of life, to bring it to a perfect adequation,
that the vegetable ſpirits of gold, (which now lay hidden as it
were idle, might make it of common gold, (which before it was)
gold phyloſophical and medicinable, which hauing gotten a
more perfect vegetation and ſeminal vertue, may be diſſolued into any liquor, and may communicate vnto the ſame that flowing
and balſamic perfection, or the Balſam of life, and of our nature.

And becauſe we are now ſpeaking of the animation of gold, *The wonder-*
ful effects of
potable gold.
be it known for a ſurety, that the auncient Fathers and Phyloſophers ſweat and laboured much to find out the miſt. ry hereof,
that they might compound a certaine Balſamic Medicine, to
vegetate and corroborate, and by the noble adequation, and the
integritie of nature thereof to conſerue the radical Balſam, and
that Nectar of our life, in good and laudable temperament. But
indeed it is not to be wondered at, that gold being deliuered from
his mannacles and fetters, and being made ſo ſpirituall and animate, and increaſed in vertue and ſtrength, doth corroborate nature, and renue the Balſam of our nature, and doth conſerue vnto the laſt period of life. being taken in a very ſmal doſe, as in the
quantity of one or two graines.

And ſo much leſſe it is to be maruailed at, that forſomuch as
by that great adequation of temperature it doth conueniently a-
gree and communicate with our radical Balſam, it doth checke
the rule of phleame, the burning of choller, and the aduſtion of
melancholy, and by his incorruptible vertue, doth preſerue our
nature, but alſo to ouercome all the diſeaſes which belong to our
body. And ſo much the rather, in regard that the ſame Balſam of
nature that natural ſpirit, is the principal cauſe in vs, of all actions, operations, and of motions, not depending vpon temperature or mixture, but concerning the ſame, as *Galen* himſelfe is
compelled to confeſſe, ſpeaking of that our natural heat. We muſt

vnderſtand

vnderſtand (ſaith he) that *Hypocrates* calleth that, inſet heate, which we call the natiue ſpirit in euery liuing thing. Neither hath any other thing formed any liuing creature from the beginning, or increaſed it, or nouriſhed it vnto the appointed time of death, but onely this inſet or natural heate, which is the cauſe of all natural workes.

Therefore they can be excuſed by no maner of meanes, which contumeliouſly, & without any reaſon, doe diſpiſe, diſcommend, and caluminat theſe kind of remedies, which doe principally tend to the reſtoring & corroborating of our radieal Balſam which alone (holpen with the ſaid medicine) is able to ſeperate thoſe things which are vnkindly & grieuous to nature, & meerely heterogenial, by expulſions conuenient, & ordinary euacuations & to retaine the homogenial & kindly parts, with the which it doth moſt eſpecially agrée to their further conſeruation. Whereas, if for the corroborating of mans ſtrength, there could bee any vſe made of leaſe gold (the which is nothing elſe but a certaine dead matter, in no ſort fit to participate with our nature, & much leſſe able to be digeſted by our natural heat) which is moſt commonly in vſe in all reſtoring medicins, as in *Confectione alkermes, electuario de gemmis, aurea Alexandrina, Diamargariton Aricennæ*, and in ſuch other like: why I pray you is the vſe of gold animate diſallowed, preſcribed in that maner and forme already ſhewed: But in good ſooth, they doe in vaine & too vnaduiſedly diſcommend, & contemptuouſly ſpeake againſt metallick remedies, as if they were no better then poyſons: when as the world knoweth, that men which are irrecouerably diſeaſed, when no other common medicines wil helpe, are then ſent to *Bathes*, to the *Spawe*, and to ſuch other waters which are medicinable, in regard they ſpring from Niter, Allum, Uitriol, Sulphur, Pitch, Antimonie, Lead & ſuch like: all which doe participate of a ſubſtance & ſpirit metallick, which we haue found by experience, to purifie & to euacuate our bodies by all manner of euacuation, not without great profit, as we will declare more at large, when we come to ſpeake more particularly of the ſame in our books concerning the hidden nature of things, and of the miſteries of Art: In the which worke we wil

ſhew

shewe plainly and openly,the vertual qualities of thofe metallick
fpirits.And it fhal be there proued by reafon,and alfo by experience,that thofe metallick fpirits, haue the fame effects that the
forefaid medicinable waters of *Bath*, and the *Spawe*,and other
fuch like haue, which are natural and naturally hote:and there-
withal we wil fhew plainly,that fuch waters artificial,by induftry may be made at any time, and in any place, and with no
leffe commodity and profit.

Bathes and waters arti-ficial.

    There are a fort of men,which in fome meafure are to be ex-
cufed,which being old,and thinke that they know all things,are
afhamed to begin now to learne againe : but they which oppofe
themfelues obftinately, and through enuy and malice,doe carpe
and cauil, are more out of courfe, againft whom we haue nothing to fay in our defence but this,that they betray their groffe
ignorance and malice.

    But the order and maner of preparing the Medicine, where-
of we treat here,was in old time called mineral, in regard that
the Philofophical Sulphur or Salt,which ferueth for animation
or vegetation, is extracted out of the firft vegetatiue fpring of
mineral nature.

    Many Philofophers haue taken Saturn or Lead for the
mineral fubiect. Other fome haue taken the Saturnal Magnefia or Loadftone, which is the firft metallick roote, and of the
ftocke and kind of vitriol. *Ifaac Holland, Ripley,* and many other
Philofophers,haue written their workes concerning this matter,the which, forfomuch as they are extant, euery one that lift
may read them . For we haue no other purpofe in this place,
but to teach and demonftrate in plaine maner, what that Balfam radical is,and that vniuerfal medicine,fo much fpoken of by
auncient philofophers, for the conferuation of health , and for
the curing of difeafes in mans body.

    Others(among whom alfo is *Raymund Lully*) fought their
fire of nature in a vegetable , to animate gold . For this
was that which al men efpecially laboured for, to put life into
gold.

                              And

And this is the reaſon why they all ſay, that there is onely one way, and one matter, oʒ Balſamick Sulphur and of nature, which yȅldeth actiue and internal fire to the ſame woʒk.

And among all vegetables, the chiefeſt is wine. Foʒ of all other it partaketh very much of the vitriolated nature: which may be gathered, not ſo much by that grȅne colloʒ of the vnripe cluſters of grapes and their ſharpe taſt as by the ſaphiric and red dy colour of thoſe that are ripe, which appeareth both within and alſo without, and by the ſharpe taſt : all which things doe plainly declare both the external and internal qualities of Vitriol.

It is alſo wel knowne that there are certaine ſuch waters in *Auuergne* in *France*, which haue the taſte of wine with a certaine pʒicking facultie oʒ reliſh.

Vineger alſo, whereto wines is eaſily bʒought, when his ſulphurus life is gone, (that is to ſay, when his ſpirit is ſeperated) doth repʒeſent the tart qualitie of Vitriol, as doth alſo other impʒeſſions of wine ſufficiently known to true Phyloſophers. The *The Chymi-* which alſo may be gathered by the concoʒdance and agreement *cal miniſtries* which wine hath with the metallick nature, ſȅing that as well out of wine as out of Vitriol, the Menſtrue of *Chymical* Art may be pʒepared, which is able to diſſolue metals into liquoʒ.

Theſe are (I ſay) the reaſons why *Raymund Lully*, and other famous Phyloſophers, placed their woʒkings in wine, foʒ the extracting of their Balſamick Sulphur, that thereby they might make true potable gold, and the infallible Balſamick medicine.

But now we wil goe foʒward to open in few woʒds *Lullies* method, which he ſo greatly did in his boke of Quinteſſence, and in other places, which if it be rightly vnderſtood, it wil eaſily direct and inſtruct euery true Phyloſopher, to extract out of all *Balſam is in* things (and therefoʒe to compound) that Balſamick medicine. *euery thing.* Foʒ the ſcope is euery where all one, there is but one ende, and there is but one onely way, to the compoſition of that Balſam oʒ Phyloſophical Sulphur, which exiſteth in all things, mineral, vegetable, and animal : howbeit in ſome moʒe, in other ſome leſſe.

CHAP.

CHAP. V.

By what Art the Sulphur and Mercury of the Phylofophers may be prepared out of a vegetable, to
make true potable gold.

Herefoze to the end all things may be duly *The fpirit of* perfozmed, which are required to fuch woz- *wine.* king, choyfe muft be made of the beft red wine that can be gotten, being made of that wine whofe wood is all fo red, and of this wine muft bee taken one hogs-head at the leaft, out of the which thou fhalt extract an *Aqua vitæ,* accozding to the woonted maner, the which thou fhalt rectifie to the higheft perfection. This fpirit of wine thou fhalt fet vp in a moft cold place, in a veffel very clofe ftopt, leaft that it bzeath out, by reafon of the exceeding fubtilty thereof. The re-mainder of the wine thou fhalt diftill againe, and there wil come out of the fame a middle *Aqua Vitæ,* if the wine bee of the beft fozt. The which fo diftilled, keepe apart, oz by it felfe. This thou fhalt doe againe with the reft of the wine, feperating as afoze the *Aqua Vitæ* from his fleame, every one feverally reftrained by it felfe. At the laft thou fhalt gather the fozces which remaine in the bottom, out of the which thou fhalt dzawe the laft humi-dutie, by a Balneum vapozofum, oz by moyft Balneum, oz by a-fhes, vntil it waxe thick and pyththie. Thefe pitchy remainders being put into divers alembicks (if they be much) put fo much thereto of the referved fleame, as may ftand aboue it foure oz fiue fingers thicke: Put altogether vpon a hote Balme, oz vp-pon hote afhes: fo within fewe dayes, the fleame which afoze was white, receiving tincture againe, will become very red,

R   hauing

hauing attracted vnto it a combustible Sulphur, out of the impure feces oz lees of the wine.

Seperate this tincted fleame by inclination, and kéepe it by it selfe if you will, foz such vses as hereafter shall bee shewed.

After that againe powze a newe quantitie of fleame vppon the same feces, in seueral allembickes, if there be great plenty of them, as is shewed afoze: that which is tincted with red, seperate againe as afoze, and powze it to that which is already tincted and seperated.

Thou shalt continue this so often, vntill the fleame will dzawe no moze rudenesse with it, and that the feces are now become somewhat white, oz Chzistalline. The which that thou maiest the moze easily knowe, powze vpon it an other fleame, and with thy finger oz a cleane sticke stirre them together, that thereby thou mayest sée whether any moze tincture remaineth. Foz all must bée cleane extracted, that the least fleame being powzed vpon it, will tinct oz colour no moze. By which pzoofe thou shalt certainly know, that the residence is very well depured, which in another place wée will call the Chzystal of tartar: because out of all common lees, and by a moze easie method, the like chzistalls are extracted.

The Christal of Tartar.

This is a most pleasant and swéete remedy, and if any in the wozld bée acceptable it is this. It doth very readily clense the stomack, the liuer and the spléene from their impurities, pzouoking vzine, and mouing one oz two sieges extraozdinarily. But let vs returne to our wozke.

The good effects of the spirit of wine.

The feces afozesaide being now rightly and conueniently pzepared and depured as is saide, must bee put into diuers smal cucurbits with long neckes, and into euery one of them, put of the rectified spirit of wine, so much, as that it may stand ouer it thzée fingers thicke: pzesently set vppon euery one of them a smal cappe oz couer, with his receiuer, strongly and well luted, *Hermetically* clo-

sed

led rounde about , that nothing breathe through : then ſet them vppon the hote aſhes that they may boyle , and diſtill : powring in againe the ſame which ſhall diſtill forth, and ſo let them boyle againe . After that ſuffer all to coole.

Then as warily as thou canſt by inclination, ſeperate the ſpirit , that nothing thick or troubled paſſe forth therewith . And then againe, powre into euery cucurbittel another ſpirit of wine, and doe as thou diddeſt afore . This thou ſhalt doe ſo often , and continue it , vntill the feces which by their owne proper nature are calcined , beginne to waxe blacke and to ſmoake , if they be put vpon a red hote plate. For this is a ſigne, that the firſt Phyloſophycall calcination is finiſhed, and that the ſpirit, by the ſame worke, is now become animate by reaſon of the tarte Balſam, and Ferment of nature, contained in the foreſaid feces , reduced into Chriſtal, as is ſaid.

Theſe animated ſpirits ioyned together, and very well reſerued, that they breathe not, nor iſſue forth, thou ſhalt put the foreſaide feces into veſſels which are called Matrats, like vnto round globes, hauing ſtraite neckes, by which the matter is powred in.

Theſe veſſels being *Hermetically* cloſed, and ſtopt, that nothing may vapour forth, let them bee couered in ſand, in the Furnace of *Athaner* , which will yeelde flame, round about the compaſſe of the foreſaide veſſell. Then put fire thereunto by the continuance of fiue or ſixe dayes , vntill the earth doe become as white as ſnowe , and is well calcined and fixed . The which , that thou maieſt make the more volatil or flying, and maieſt alſo make the Sulphur and Mercury of the Phyloſophers, thou mayeſt if thou wilt diuide this thy callixe into two or three cucurbittils of conuenient greatneſſe, firſt waighing the waight of euery of the calxes, and powring vpon euery of them a forth part of the ſpirit of wine, animated as aforeſaide.

Put

B. M. figuifi-
eth Balneum
maria.

Put a fmal head vpon each of the cucurbittels, with their fe-
ucral receiuers wel fitted as afoze. Place them in B. M. which
is moyft, by the fpace of one day: After that, the fame veffels being fet in afhes, put thereto a meane fire that the liquoz may
diftill fozth, which whereas afoze it was moft ardent and moft
fharpe, now it fhal come fozth altogether without tafte, hauing
no other relifh vppon the tongue and palat, then hath common
wel-water : the reafon hereof is, foz that the fozefaid fpirit, hath
left and fozfaken his Balfamic Salt, which afoze being mixed
with the fpirit ftilled fozth with the Salt of the fozefaid Calx: Foz
nature loueth nature, and followeth her in her nature, as Phylofophers teach.

Then againe thou fhalt powze on another fpirit of wine
animate, as afoze, in the fame pzopoztion, and the foz-
mer ozder of diftillation obferued, vntill in tafte thou finde
the fozefaide animate fpirit, to come fozth and to diftil, as
ftrong in tafte and relifh, as it was then when thou powzedft it
on.

Foz this fhall be a figne, that the fozefaide fixed Salt, hath
retained out of the volatil, fo much as fhal be fufficient and conuenient to retaine.

And now if thou waigh and counterpoyfe thy matters, thou
fhalt finde that they are increafed a third part in waight :
as if there were one ounce in euery veffell of Calxe, thou
fhalt finde that euery of them doth waigh thzee ounces oz
moze.

The which is diligently to bee obferued foz fublimation,
and foz the laft wozking which as yet refteth to bee done
that the volatill may tranfcende, and ouercome the fixed.

In the which bufineffe that thou maieft pzocede the
moze fafely, thou muft take fome of the fozefaide Phylofo-
phycal Calxe vine, and caft it vppon a red hote plate of
yzon, and if thou fee all the faide Calxe to vapour away and
to banifh in fmoake, like Salarmoniack, thou haft an abfolute
and

and perfect worke. If otherwise, thou must begin the foresaide worke againe, and continue it, vntil the foresaid signe doe appeare.

This done, thou shalt put these matters into smal long Lymbeckes in forme of a Sublimatorie, with heads vpon them, and receiuers to receiue the spiritual sulphurus humiditie: and then thou shalt distil it in ashes with a gentle fire, by the space of a whole day: afterward thou shalt increase the fire by a further degree, more & more, so long, vntil about the end of eighteene houres or twenty, the fire bee made sublimatorie, and that thou see the vessels to bee no more obscured or darkened with spirites: or with white fumes. And then shal yee see the sublimated matter cleauing to the sides of the glasses, fayre and bright, and transparent like vnto pearles, or such like. Vppon this matter beaten into powder, in a Purphorie morter of smal bignesse, thou shalt powder the sulphurus spirit distilled, moystening it by little and little, and boyling or straining the whole by the space of foure dayes in a strong Athanor.

And thus thou shalt haue a pearelike matter, a Balsam radical, extracted from a Uegetable, the Mercurie of the Philosophers, the Sulpur Balsamick, and to conclude, that fire of Nature so much commended, and so hidden by al the Philosophers, which with one consent say, *Ignis & azoc tibi sufficient*: Let Fire, and the Matter suffice thee. *A Balsam Radicai.*

This onely Balsam is the vniuersal medicine, to defend and conserue health, if it be giuen with some conuenient liquor to the quantitie of one or two graines. Great and admirable is the vertue thereof, to restore our radical Balsam: the which wee affirme to be the Medicine of diseases, euen by the common consent of al Physitians.

But our *Lullie* and other Philosophers, are not content with this, but proceeding further, do dissolue the forsaid Philosophical Sulphur in a conuenient portion of the spirit of wine, rectified to perfection, as afore, and suffer them to be vnited, and very well coupled together by way of Circulation in a Pellican Hermetically stopt or closed: and within fewe dayes, the water

is made azure like oz Celestial: which being distilled, is of soze
to dissolue gold, and doth reduce it into the true Calxe of the
Phylosophers, into a pzecious liquoz, which itterated circulations and distillations, can also passe by the necke of the Allembic
oz by Retozt.

In the which wozking, if thou pzocéde as thou shouldst, thou
shalt be able to separate from gold (already phylosophically dissolued and animated) thy phylosophical dissoluing, which wil
continually serue foz newe dissolutions. Foz very little is left

Potable gold, in euery dissolution. And so thou hast the true potable golde:
the vniuersal Medicine, which neuer can bé valued béing in-
estimable, noz yet sufficiently commended.

After the same manner thou shalt make the dissolutions of
Pearles, and of pzetious stones, most general remedies, and de-
seruing to be placed among the chiese, if they bé dissolued after
the ozder and manner afozesaid, with a natural dissoluing. Remedies J say, which can much better confirme and strengthen
our nature, than if accozding to the common manner, they bé
onely powdzed and searced, as is wont to bé done in those our
common pzeparations and cozdial powders.

But some paraduenture wil say, that these kinde of pzeparations are too hard, oz such as they vnderstand not, oz at least care
not to vnderstand.

But this is a vaine obiection to pzeuent foz excuse of their ig-
nozance, the difficultie of these pzeparations, and the pzotract of
time, when as the thing is neither difficile, noz long, to them
which know how to take it in hand. These things are not to bé
estéemed, noz labour is to bé spared, to attaine so excellent & pzecious medicine, which in so little & smal a dose, as in the quantitie of one oz two graines, can wozke so great and wonderful effects: which bzingeth great commendation and honour to the
Physitian, and to the sicke perfect health and vnspeakable sollace
and ioy.

But to conclude, J wil say with *Cicero,* in his *Tusculans:*
*There is no measure of seeking after the truth : and to be wearie
of seeking, is disgrace, whē that which is sought for is most excellent.*
C A HP.

CHAP. VI.

The way to prepare and make the Balſamick Medicine, out of all things.

Y the foreſaid preparation of ſulphur, Bal-ſamick vegetable, which wée haue before taught, faithfully, plainly, and manifeſtly, it is eaſie to vnderſtand, after what manner the ſame Sulphur may bée extracted out of euery mixed body. In the wich bodie (that I may ſummarily gather al things toge-ther) there is firſt found a liquor, without al odour, or relliſhing taſte, which is called Phlegme, or paſſiue water. Then commeth a liquor which hath taſte, colour, odour, and other impreſſions of vertual qualities, which is called the Mercurial liquor. And after that commeth forth an oylie liquor, which floteth aloft, and conceuing flame, which is cal-led Sulphur.

1. Phlegme.
2. Mercury.
3. Sulphur.

After the extraction of theſe thrée ſeueral moyſtures, there remaineth nothing but aſhes, or dry part: out of the which aſhes, béeing wel calcined, Salt is extracted, with his proper Phlegme, melſhing oftentimes, and powring water warmed, vpon the foreſaid aſhes, put into *Hypocrates* bagge, and repea-ting this ſo often times, til you perceiue a Salt water to come, which hath a briniſh taſte: after the ſame manner, as women are wont to make their lye-waſh.

4. Salt.

This béeing done, let the moyſt be diſtilled, and the ſalt wil remaine in the bottome. The which ſalt notwithſtanding, in this firſt preparation is not made cleane enough, nor ſufficiently pu-rified. Wherefore the ſame diſtilled water is to be powred vp a-gaine, that the Salt may againe bée diſſolued in the ſame: the which ſo diſſolued, filter it, or ſtraine it through a bag oftentimes, as afore, til it be moſt cleare: then coagulate it at a gentle heate. And after this maner thou mayſt extract a Salt, cleare & pure, out

of

of al vegetable afhes. Uppon this Salt being put into an Allembic, powze al his mercurial fharpe water: let them be digefted
by the fpace of one oz two dayes, in the gentle heate of the
Balme: and then let them be diftilled by afhes, and fo the water
wil diftil fozth without tafte oz rellifh.   Becaufe whatfoeuer it
contained of the volatile Salt, wil refide in the bottome with his
per fired falt. Goe fozward therefoze in thy wozking as befoze I
taught thee concerning the wine.

Oz if thou wilt not wozke fo exactly, melhe vp againe al the
mercurial liquoz, and make it paffe thzough the fozefaid Salt,
which wil take into it, al that vitriol impzeffion which that water fhal haue, and the water oz liquoz, fhal haue neither rellifh noz
tafte, but fhal be altogether like to common water. But if thou
adde fo much that the volatile part doe exceed the fired, that is to
fay, that there be moze of the volatile, than of the fired, (the which
thou fhalt eafily know by waight, becaufe it wil be increafed
thzeefold, oz by trial vpon a red hote copper oz Iron plate, when
this matter being caft vppon the fame, vapoureth and paffeth
away in fmoke) then thou moft fublime it, and it wil become the
Sal Armoniack of the Philofophers: (fo it pleafeth them to cal
this matter) which wil bee cleare and tranfparant like pearles.

Uppon this powozed matter, thou fhalt powze by little and
litle the oylie liquoz purified, and thou fhalt boyle this matter,
that of volatil it may be fired againe. Neuerthelefle, that which
fhal be fired, fhal be of nature moze fufible than waxe, and con-
fequences wil moze eafily communicate with fpirits and with
our natural Balfam, when it is feperated from his paffiue water, and paffiue earth which are vnpzofitable.

Both which matters the Phylofophers cal the paffiue Element, becaufe they containe no pzopertie in them, neither doe
they fhew fozth any action. And thus a body oz nature is made
wholely homogenical & fimple: albeit there are to bee feene, thzee
diftinct natures, the which notwithftanding are of one oz the
fame effence and nature.

And fo a body fhal bee compounded exactly pure out of thofe
thzee hypoftatical beginnings, namely falt, Mercurie, and Sulphur.

Elements
paffiue.

phur. The which Sulphur in ſome part is anſwerable to
truely ſimple, and Elementarie fire: Mercurie, to Ayre and
to Water: in like manner moſt ſimply and truely Elementarie: and Salt, to pure Earth, ſimple and Elementarie. The which Earth is not colde and dead, but hote
earth, liuing earth, and full of actiue, and vegetable qualities. *Actiue Ele-*
ments.

Beholde then how a perfect and vniuerſall Medicine is prepared out of all the things of Nature. The which it thou
wilt vſe for purgation, chooſe for thy ſubiect ſome purging ſimple, if thou wilt, eſpecially corroborate and ſtrengthen, make
choiſe of ſuch things as doe yeelde moſt comfort. If thou wilt
either ſpecially or generally lenifie, and mittigate paine, then
chooſe ſuch things as are moſt lenifying and aſſwagers of
paine.

And yet know thou this, that in one and the ſame Remedie
onely, prepared in this manner, as for example, in the nature of Balſamick Salt, thou haſt a clenſer and a purger, and
an vniuerſal emptier, a corrector of all impurities and corruptions.

Thou haſt alſo in the particular nature of Sulphur, a general and ſpiritual anodine or aſſwager. In the Mercurial na- *A Medicine*
ture, there is an vniuerſal comfortatiue and the ſame nouriſhing: *particular*
Al which natures ioyned together as afore, by the Art and in- *and general.*
duſtrie of a true Phyſition and Phyloſopher, are able to performe and effect al theſe functions, without any griefe and perturbation: and in the meane time it doth corroborate by
his Balſamical vertue or radical Balſam, ſupplying vnto it
al meanes, not onely for defence, but alſo for expulſion and ſup-
preſſion of al diſeaſes.

And this is the true Medicine, this is the reaſon of his vniuer-
ſalitie, this is his puritie and perfection.

Neither is there any thing more eaſie then the preparation
thereof, if it be rightly vnderſtood. Moreouer, ſo exceeding great
is the vtillitie and excellencie thereof, that no labour, no
paines, no induſtrie, ought to bee omitted, or to bee repu-

S   ted

ted hard, whatfoeuer difficultie oz doubts may arife, oz bæ obiected.

But if there bæ any man, which wil not take vpon him this labour, albeit moſt pzofitable, and ozdained foz health and the pzolonging of mans life, and foz the fame bæ may exactly pzepare thefe Ballamick medicines : yet at the leaſt hee wil by the meanes thereof, as it were by a certaine Directoz, ſéke out in general, the euacuating, mundifying, and clenfing faculties, which are in moſt vfe, and which chiefly confiſt in Salts : and in like manner the aſſwagers, mittiga-tozs, and healers, in Sulphur and Oile : and finally the nou-rifhers, reſtozers, and comfozters in the liquoz oz Mer-curie.

And by the fame way and reafon it ſhal bæ taught, that the true cozrectozs of all remedies, are purifying and cocti-ons only: and that thefe alone are the true hony and Sugar, to ſwæten al things.

Foz thofe things alfo which are moſt tart, ſharpe, and fowze, yea and bitter, are by this meanes made ſwæte, and al manner of euil qualitie rozrected, and contempered, euen as fruites befoze their perfect concoction, and maturitie, are tart, ſharpe and fouze, euery one accozding to their kinde and qualitie.

So wæ ſé, that wines, in whofe maturation oz rypening the heate of the Sunne failed, are made moze crude and ſharpe: which is the reafon why fome yéeres, wines are made moze ripe, acceptable, and better agræing with nature, albeit they came as wel afoze, as then, from one vine. Albeit much hærein is to be attributed to the region alfo, and to the place, whereinto the beames of the Sunne may make a moze ſtrong impzeſſion.

The Caufe why fome wines are fweet, and fome fowre.

And this may bæ the caufe, that fome are ſwæte, and ful of wine, fome meane, others very crude,and fcarce wine.

So the Tigurine wines, and others in mountaine places, which are colde, are foz the moſt part crude ; and muſt haue a further rypening in their caſkes, befoze they can bæ dzunke with pleafure and pzofite. Alfo the fame wines wanting a
kindly

kindely rypening and concoction, remaining ftill crude, are fo full of lees, and tartarous matter, that the inhabitants which dwell in thofe places, where thefe wines doe growe, *Crude wines* are moze fubiect to the difeafe of the Stone, than others. *breede the*

Now, if this defect bee to bee fame in wine, fo greatly nutri- *ftone.* tiue, and agreeing with our nature: what fhall wee fay of *Hellebor*, and of many other poifonfull Medicines which fpzing out of moft colde Mountaines, and wilde, without Tillage, much leffe are they concocted by the Moone?

Therefore no maruaile that our *Hellebor* anfwereth not *Hellebore* thofe effects, which *Hypocrates* attributeth vnto it. For that *poifonfull.* which he commendeth in *Greece*, commeth out of a conuenient Region, where no doubt there are Plants and Wines of greater efficacie. Wherefore I haue vfed foz a firft pzeparati- on of *Hellebors*, to tranfplant them into gardens, fcituate in a moze temperate foyle and place.

The which how much they differ from thofe which grow *Tranfplan-* vpon wild and cold mountaines, as do alfo garden Succoze and *ting of herbs* endiue, from the wylde, the difference and vfe, doe fufficiently *helpeth their* declare. *nature.*

But thofe pzeparations, which pzoceede and are done by Art, and the concoctions which Art imitating nature fini- fheth, are much better, and moze contracted and fweetned, as by the pzeparation following, farre moze exact than that thofe common, in which there appeareth nothing but that which is crude and impure, fhal manifeftly appeare, and the thing it felfe plainely pzoue.

P 2 C A HP.

CHAP. VII.

The vertue, and preheminence of the Medicine Balſamick.

Ome Phyloſophers ſæke the matter of Medicine in our ſelues : otherſome in the bony of the animal and Celeſtial nature : otherſome in a certain animal nature, not in act o₂ effect, but in power : which repreſenteth the ſimilitude of the wo₂ld, and which conteineth in his belly Gold and ſiluer, white and red : Sulphur, and Mercury : which Nature the moſt ancient diſpoſer vnder God, hath mixed together by due p₂opo₂tion. Out of the which matters, by ſund₂y ſay₂e and long p₂eparations, they p₂epared their vniuerſal Medicine : which by reaſon of perfect contemperance, adequation, and puritie, can contemperate, conſerue, and alſo increaſe the radical humour, and that quickening Nectar of ours: becauſe in puritie of his ſpiritual nature, hæ doth communicate with our ſpirits.

Furthermo₂e, let vs ſæ how much the ſaid Medicine perfo₂meth in the d₂iuing away diſeaſes, and what infinite multitude of remedies it hath. And firſt, ſe₂ſomuch as it may be applyed and fitted to al intentions requiſitie (as may be gathered by that which hath bæne ſaid afo₂e) and ſo₂ſomuch as it may bæ giuen in ſo ſmall a doſe, which wil b₂ing no violent action, no₂ loathſomneſſe to our body, no₂ any kind of perturbation, and yet neuertherleſſe wo₂keth excæding wel, acco₂ding to the diſpoſition of our nature, I ſæ no reaſon why this vniuerſal and moſt noble Medicine, ſhould not be p₂eferred befo₂e theſe rapſodies of Medicines.

Who ſo vſeth rightly this Medicine; and in fit time, ſhal bæ refreſhed and co₂robo₂ate, and ſo armed with ſtrength, that from thencefo₂th hæ ſhal mo₂e eaſily and readily ſhake off

Hermeticall Phyficke.

off his fickneffe : whereof nature otherwife being deftitute, would eafily be ouercome. Let vs vfe a familiar example that thofe things which we haue hitherto fpoken, may moꝛe plainly appeare to all men.

Wee fee in our elementall fire,that if thou caft into the fame a-ny thing that wil eafily take flame, as ftrawe,oꝛ any fuch thing which wil readily burne and increafe the foꝛce of burning,which befoꝛe was almoft extinguifhed,foꝛ becaufe it was deftitate as it were of nourifhment,and wholy as it were ouerwhelmed of af-fhes: So alfo our radicall Balfam the fire bꝛand , and burning lampe of the fire of our nature, wanting conuenient and pꝛoper nourifhment whereby it fainteth,oꝛ elfe fo ouerwhelmed by the feces and afhes of obftructions,that it is in danger of fuffocation and fmothering,oꝛ elfe hindꝛed by fome other caufe,whereby it cannot exercife liuing flame foꝛ the conferuation of our life:then indeed it ftandeth in neede of a calefactoꝛ, and reftoꝛer of heate, that in better maner and moꝛe readily it may fhew foꝛth the pꝛo-per qualities and functions . The like reafon and confideration alfo is to be had concerning our natural Balfam, the which being diminifhed , oꝛ being hindꝛed oꝛ hurt by any occurrent outwardly,being againe increafed by that Balfamick medicine, it arifeth eft foone , and moft perfectly perfoꝛmeth his wonted functions. Foꝛ feeing that medicinall Balfam is of a certaine e-thereal nature oꝛ a heauenly fire,becaufe it quickeneth and bur-neth not, noꝛ confumeth: therefoꝛe out of hand, as if it were a permanent and certaine fpirituall water of life, it doth commu-nicate,and is as it were vnited with our fpirit,and doth repaire and increafe it,by reafon of the fimpathy,and common likeneffe therewith. Neither is it to be thought,that this commeth fo to paffe,foꝛ any other caufe,but only of this (as was faid euen now) namely of that friendly conuenience , and agræing friendfhip, which that Balfamick medicine,hath with our radical Balfam. The which is the onely reafon why I call the one , Balfam of life, and the other the medicinal Balfam , euen foꝛ the relatiue conuenience of them both. And yet befide this fimilitude and fa-miliarity of nature,it hath other particular vertues. Foꝛ it is en-

duced

dued with great actiuitie, it is fpiritual and exceeding pearcing. for this caufe it doth attenuate and make thinne, it doth digeft, diffolue, and euacuate thefe feculent ftuffings and afhes, threatening peril of fuffocation and choaking to the Balfam of life. Moreouer, if there be any impurity or corruption, by which it is much offended, by what other meanes can it bee more fafely and better rooted out, then by a thing fo pure and incorruptible? And if any burning feauer doe inuade the body and the inftrumental parts of life about the heart, with what more conuenient Sharpe Syrup, or Syrup of Limons, canft thou extinguifh it, then by the Balfamick fharpneffe of this our medicine? Let gun-poulder fpeake for vs ; and by a fufficient teftimony of this thing, which this liquor doth not onely extinguifh, but alfo will not fuffer it to take flame, but maketh it idle. Witneffes alfo are the moft burning and volatil fpirits, which al the Ife of the Northerne mountaines cannot congeale, and yet are congealed with that liquor in *Balneo Mariæ*: yet with all, the fame liquor hath this property, that it wil attemperate and diffolue the moft hard Ife. Is there any paine and griefe that would be affwaged? This medicine fhal be thy mittigating anodine, and moft healthfome Nepenthes. Is there any peftilent poyfon, or malignant quality to be extyrped? There is not a more fafe Treacle or Mithridate then this, which is the fumme of all Alexipharmacons, & the moft chiefe preferuatiue from all infection. Is the heart to be corroborated, & the fpirits to be vegetated? No confection Alkermes, no confection of Hyacinth is to be preferred before this balfam. To conclude, what more fpeedy altering medicine can there be found, which is able to correct a diftemperature, then that moft temperat remedy? To thefe vnfpeakeable vertues, adde yet this one, that this medicine, neuer bringeth with it a glutting loathfomneffe, or perturbation of the body: but quickly, fafely, & pleafantly performeth his workings. And the fame with fo fmall a doe, that whereas in other medicine, ounces, are required, in this a few graines diffolued in wine or in broath, or in other conuenient liquor, are fufficient to be oppofed againft the ficknee, which produce great and wonderful effects.

Thefe

is vnprofitable and vaine. For nature is alwaies one and like to her selfe, neither is she at any time idle in vs, but is perpetually occupied, alway stirring, mouing, and vegetating, vntill by too much let, she being hindred, shee doe worke more slowly and weakely. The which impediments and contrarieties, she her selfe of her owne accorde, and by her owne proper strength goeth about to put away and ouercome: But when she hath to doe with a most strong enemie, or with many, she sooner and far more easily can ouercome them, if she be strengthened with the helpes of arte, and hauing conuenient meanes, she shall with greater strength and security preuaile.

To bring which thing to passe, our Balsamick medicine by that exquisite preparation, hath gotten a most pure, quickening, spiritual, strengthening, and kindly nature, which without all exception, is farre more conuenient and effectual, then other medicines of common Physitians, prepared by no arte, by no industry, or dexterity.

The which, forsomuch as they are yet crude, impure, and grosse, and are clogged with a terrestrial thicknesse, they doe rather cloy and ouerlay nature, before she can extract their maligne quality, concoct their cruditie, and deuide their earthly grossnesse and impurity: the which being her taske and burden, shee fainteth before shee can receiue any helpe or comfort.

And that we may not digresse from our similitude, let vs apply that which is said, to fire, whereof we haue spoken before. As we see fire when it is ouerwhelmed with many ashes, and hindred from taking aier, (by which it is nourished) is easily smothered and put out: and that the same againe is stirred vp, if a man with his hand doe rake away the ashes, and doe blowe the sparkes which remaine, giuing free accesse of the aier: heers the cause of the fires refreshing and beginning againe, is attributed to him which remoued the Ashes, when as indeede hee was but the instrument of restoring the fire.

But the principal efficient consisteth in the fire it selfe, the which he had spread abroad and winded or bellowed in vaine,

L   ij if it had bene quite and cleane out. Wherefore that renuing is to be attributed to the fire alone which remained as to the first, nert, and infet caufe, onely the outward ventilation or winding conuning betwéene as the inftrument.

Moreouer, as we fée, that when the fire is fo weake, that very fewe fparkes are to bee found, that then in vaine a great heape of dead coales are caft vpon the fame to make a fpédy fire, which will fooner put altogether out, then make a quick fire.

But if thou put vpon them quicke burning coales, they will by and by increafe the fire, without feare of extinction: euen fo in like maner, the principal vertue or function, is alway to be afcribed to our vital or radical Balfam, rather then to the Phyfition or Medicine, albeit the fame may bee fome helpe, in putting away the affie feces, and in t diffoluing the troubled lées which are an impediment, that fo it may more fréely haue tranfpiration and aire, that by them it be not oppreffed and choaked.

Such is this Balfamick Medicine, which being purified, exalted, and brought vnto the higheft effence and perfection, it doth ftirre vppe, refrefh, and reftore our vitall fire, lining, but yet languifhing, to his former vigor and ftrength. The which, forfomuch as it doth fooner, more fafely, and more pleafantly performe without all comparifon then that other ordinary and common Phyfick; thou fhalt not mifcompare that of theirs to dead coales, or to gréene wood, but this of ours as prepared and brought to a Balfam, to a burning coale, which is the fumme of our whole difputation.

Let thefe things fuffice to be fpoken concerning the property, quality, & excellency of our Balfamick medicine, which Phylofophers prepare out of one thing onely, not out of many, whether it be mineral, vegetal, or animal. Of this medicine alone is the Syrach,38.4 faying of the wife man to be vnderftood, when he faith; The Lord hath created medicine out of the earth, and he that is wife wil not abhorre it. For by this word (Medicine) he vnderftandeth remedy

remedy, not the Art of Phyſick. For it was ordinary and common in thoſe firſt ages, to vſe this medicine, taken out of one onely matter. But the latter age ſuccæding, after long ſearch, found out that radical Balſam, and ſaw by experience, that it was in ſome thing more; and in other ſome leſſe. Whatſoeuer it is, it is knowne that they of olde time did vſe moſt ſimple remedies: neither did they care for ſo great confuſion of compoſitions and mixtures which fill a whole ware-houſe and ſhoppe, as our Phyſitians and Apothecaries do at this day.

And if we will conſider of thoſe things which *Theophraſtus Dioſcorides*, and others of the auncients haue left vnto vs in writing, concerning medicine, and the vertues of ſimple remedies, we ſhal perceiue and finde, that they vſed the moſt ſimple method and order of curing, and that they had not ſo much reſpect to the actiue or paſſiue qualities, of hote and cold, of dry and moyſt, out of the which came the originall of ſo many mixtions and confuſions. But it is plaine and euident, that they attributed to their ſimples, this and that property, either becauſe they had ſo learned from others, peraduenture by tradition, or elſe by experience, obſeruing the impreſſions, formes, and figures of their ſimples.

But they of more late time haue bene ſo raſh of iudgement, that they wil take vpon them to iudge of the faculties of ſimples by their taſte and reliſh, and thereby diſcerne and determine, their firſt, ſecond, and third qualities, to the which afterward all the vertue of the ſaide ſimples was attributed. But becauſe they found not this an vniuerſal rule alwaies and in all things, and that it did deceiue, therefore ſome fled to the ſecret and hidden properties, aryſing from the forme, and the whole ſubſtance.

Theſe and ſuch like ſtarting holes and ſubtilties, haue brought vpon vs great incertainty and doubtfulneſſe, which way to diſcerne and find out thoſe things, which ſerue for our beſt good.

Tell me I pray you (if you can) how many bitter things

there are in taſte, which neuertheleſſe according to the edict of that rule, are not hote at all? Of this ſort among others many moe is Opium and Cichory. Againe, how many ſowre things are there, which by their rule ſhould be moſt cold, which notwithſtanding are moſt hote, as the ſpirits of Uineger of Niter, and of Sulphur? How many ſweet things are there in outward taſte, which in their internal ſubſtance are nothing at all contempered. How many things are outwardly and at the firſt beginning of taſte, altogether vnſauory and without reliſh, which inwardly and in faculty, are moſt ſharpe and byting. Honey, Caſſia, and Sugar, are in their internal ſubſtance ſo hote and violent, that out of them alſo may be prepared ſuch diſſoluers, as are wont to be made out of Aqua Fortis, or Aqua Regalis: which can diſſolue gold and ſiluer as ſpeedily as the other.

A Diſſoluing water.

Lead yeeldeth out no taſte to the tongue: and yet his internall ſubſtance, is a certaine ſugared delightfull ſweeteneſſe. So outwardly Copper hath no reliſh and is of a ruddie colour: but that greene where into it is changed, is moſt ſharpe.

Copper is red without and greene within.

We might ſhewe of ſuch examples, almoſt an infinit number, whereunto we muſt not raſhly giue credit, nor ſtand vpon taſte, nor leane to much vpon the exteriour qualities and temperament of things. For if they be more inwardly and exactly examined, then by that ſuperficiary and ſlight maner of taſting and experimenting, and that heir inward bowels, be diligently anatomized, they ſhal be found farre otherwiſe, and oftentimes different, not onely in taſte, but alſo in odour, in colour, and in their whole ſubſtance.

But if ſo be a ſeperation be made of the three hypoſtaticall or ſubſtantial eſſential beginnings, as of Salt, Sulphur, and Mercury, then there will appeare a true and lawfull difference of taſtes. Becauſe one and the ſame ſubſtance may containe in it ſeuerall taſtes. How then canſt thou giue a ſafe iudgement of his properties and vertues? As for example, conſider well of *Guaiacum*: whoſe diuers vertues and properties therein contained, thou canſt not eaſily diſcerne by ſimple taſte.

Neither

Neither canst thou alleage any certaine cause why it should be *Diaphoretical*, that is to say, apt to prouoke sweates: which by the separation of the aforesaid beginnings, thou canst attaine vnto. For thou shalt find in his mercurial tartnesse, & in his oylie sulphurus, and thinner substance, that facultie to enforce sweate, which is also in Juniper, in Bore, in Oake, in Ashe, and almost in al woodes and barkes, as also in many other things: but here-after wee wil shewe the cause, why those sharpe and sulphurus substances, doe prouoke sweates. But you may also extract out of the same bitterish *Guaiacum*, a Salt apt for purgation, and euacuation of humours. The like is to bee said of *Cinamom*, and almost of all other things. For *Cinamom* hath facultie both to bind and to loose. The opening force consisteth in his sulphu-rus oilie, and thinne substance, which being separated from his feces, thou shalt find a substance of the nature of *Allum*, won-derfully binding.

Also whereas Opium is bitter. that commeth by reason of his Salt, from the which being separated by his oile or narcoti-cal Sulphur, it becommeth purging no lesse than out of any other bitter thing, as if out of *Gentian Centorie*, & such like, the same Salt should bee separated and rightly prepared. *Narcotical is Stupefac-tiue.*

To these bitter Salts is giuen the name of *Salt-gemme* as a difference of other Saltes, whereof there is great diuersitie of kindes, as more at large shall be shewed in another place. But nowe in fewe wordes I say, that some Saltes are bitter, some sweete, some tart, sowre, sharpe, austere, pricking, and brinish: whose particular facultie, is rightly attributed to the proper sub-stance of the same Salt, rather than to any other qualitie, what-soeuer the same be.

THE THIRD PART OF THIS

Worke: wherein is contained a fmall Treatife, *concerning the Seales and Impreſsions of things,* by Hermeticall Philofophers, with much care, and fingular diligence, gathered and brought to light.

Ll men follow not one way to attaine to a generall knowleoge of all things. The way of the Empericks is vncertaine, fo that it is traceo in the darkeneſſe of ignorance. Theſe haue reſpect to the external impreſſions, and to fome fuſet qualitites, eſpecially to thofe which map be ſeen, tafted, and ſmelt. Furthermore, they haue great regard to the firſt qualities, hote, cold moyſt and dzie: which they haue made the beginnings and firſt foundations of thefe faculties oz vertues.

But the Hermeticall Phylofophers and Chymiſts, leauing thofe bare qualities of the bodyes, fought the foundations of their actions, taſtes, odours, and colours, elfe where. At the laſt by wittie inquifition they knew that there were thzee diſtinct fubſtances in euery natural elemented body: that is to fap, Salt, Sulphur, and Mercurie. And thefe internal beginnings of things, they called hypoſtatical vertual, and ozdinatiue beginnings. For in thefe thzee hypoſtatical beginnings, thofe forefaid vertual and fenſible qualities, are to be found, not by imagination, analogie, oz coniecture, but in very deede and in effect. That is to fap, tafles in Salt, moſt chiefly: odours in Sulphur: colours out of both, but moſt chiefely out of Mercurie: becaufe

Mer-

Mercurie hath the volatile Salt of al things, ioyned vnto it. For there are two kindes of ſalts, the one fixed, the other vo-latile,as ſhal be ſhewed anon.

Therefore ſalt is firme, fixed., and ſubſtantifying begin-ning of al things : and therefore it is compared with the pure E-lement of Earth. Becauſe ſalt is not cold & dry by his owne na-ture (as it is holden of ſome that the Earth is) the which quali-ties are the death of things : but it is rather hote, and endued with an actiue qualitie, for that it is appointed to ſerue for the generation of all things.

Sulphur is compared to fire,for as fire,ſo ſulphur doth quick-ly take flame:and burne: euen as alſo do al other things, which partake of the nature thereof,ſuch as are Roſinis,fat,and oylie.

Mercurie by Analogie anſwereth the Ayre, and Water. For not only that dry minerall water, (which is alſo called Hy-drargire and Quick ſiluer) is called Mercurie: but alſo euery water or actiue liquor endued with any vertue, is alſo for the ex-cellencie thereof called Mercurie. The which Mercurie (as we haue ſaid) may bee likened to either Element, that is to ſay, to Ayre, and to Water: to Ayre,becauſe when it is put to the fire, it is found almoſt nothing but Ayre, or a vapour, which vani-ſheth away. This if you pleaſe you may call a moyſt actiue.

And it may bee compared to water alſo,becauſe it is running : and ſo long as it continueth in his owne nature, it is not con-tained in his owne liſts, but in the limmits of another : which according to Ariſtotle, is the definition of moyſt.

Theſe three beginnings, (I ſay) are found in all bodyes as internal and neceſſarie ſubſtances for the compoſition of a mixt body.

For ſeeing the foreſaid Mercurial, volatile, and ſpirituall hu-miditie, cannot eaſily be conioyned with the earthie, corporeal, and fixed part, by reaſon of that great difference and contrariety of either of them: it is neceſſarily required, that there ſhould bee a meane , and indifferent partaking of either : that is as wel of the ſpirituall as of the fixed, to conioyne both in one.

And

Sulphur the meane to ioyne salt and Mercu-rie.

And this indifferent meane is Sulphur or oile, which holdeth a meane betwæene that which is fixed, and that which is flying. For oyles, are neuer so quickly, so easily, and so wel distilled, as are waters: because the substance of Sulphur, or of an oylie bodie is tenax and retentiue, and therefore most apt to combinde the other two, to effect a good, perfect and equal mixture.

To make the matter more plaine by example. For as a man can neuer make good closing mortter, of water and sand onely, without the mixture of lime, which bindeth the other two together like oile and glue: so Sulphur or the oily substance, is the mediator of Salt and Mercurie, and coupleth them both together: neither doth it onely couple them to death, but it doth also represse and contemperate the acrimonie of Salt, and the sharpnesse of Mercurie, which is found to bée very much therein. Much like to the coniunction which the Spirite and quickening moyst radical maketh betwæene the soule, an incorporeat substance, and the body, which very much differeth from the same.

Three natures in one.

Thus then it appeareth, after what manner these thrée natures may consist in one, together, and so to be made a mixed and perfect bodie. For as salt by it selfe alone cannot bring this thing to passe: euen so neither these two fluxible and mouing humors, cannot without Salt by their nature compose a firme, fixed, and solyd body.

Moreouer Sulphur must néedes bée had as a Glue without the which the Mercurial liquor will be swallowed vp by the dryncsse of the terrestrial Salt, and through the violence of the heate of the fire, which by the Sulphur is contained. But the Mercurial humour, is as it were the chariot of the other two, seruing to penetrate, and to make the mixture easie and spædy.

If there bée any man, which through obstinacie, or blockishnesse of wit, doth not well conceiue and vnderstand this: let him beholde and consider of the blood which is in mans body, how in the same, the whaye is as a chariot or mediator, and combiner of the other two beginnings together, as may appeare by the preparation and separation thereof.

Very

Very fitly wee may vſe this example in this place. And hereafter, by infallable and euident demonſtration, we wil ſhew after what manner, the other two beginnings, beſide the whaye (which ſupplyeth the place of Mercuries) are in blood.   When Salt is predominate and beareth the ſwaye, it produceth ſo many kindes of diuers Vlcers and many other diſeaſes: beſide that portion of ſalt which paſſeth through the reines and bladder, by Vrines. In like maner we haue already ſhewed how Sulphur, or the oilie part, is in the ſame blood. This ſulphur being exalted, it cauſeth ſulphurus exhalation, as inflamatiõs, from whence come ſo many kindes of Feauers. So, Mercurial ſublimations raiſe Rheumes and Catarres, with other diſeaſes Mercurial.

Salt cauſeth Vlcers in the body.

Chymiſtes determine, that there are ſundry kindes of ſalt, which as they are found apart in nature, ſo alſo in all mixt bodyes.

That is to ſay, common ſalt (which the Sea by his ſecret Cunui pypes doth conuey through the earth:) Salt gemme alſo, Allum (whereof there are diuers kindes) Vitriol, Salt-Armoniac, and Salt Niter, which men commonly call Salt peter.

Saltes of diuers ſortes.

Among theſe ſalts, two are flying, and are mixed with liquors after an inſenſible manner: that is to ſay, Niter, & Salt-Armoniac of nature. Niter doth participate of ſulphur, and of the oylie liquor of things: Armoniac partaketh of Mercurie, or of the Mercurial humour of things.

And theſe foreſaid ſalts, (which are found both in earthie, and metallick ſubſtances) are deriued through the benefite of rootes, into hearbs plants, and trees: which becauſe they are alwayes in the earth, they retaine the nature moſt chiefly of fixed ſalt.

And after the ſame manner, the nature of fixed ſalt, is to bee ſought for in rootes. In flowers alſo and in leaues, there is great ſtore of the other two flying Salts, which being ſuch, they eaſily vaniſh away and come to nothing; when the flowers and leaues doe wyther and waxe dry. But thoſe plants and hearbes which take their nouriſhment from fixed ſalt, are alwayes kept flowriſhing and greene: and therefore they doe the more ſtrongly reſiſt the fainting heate of Sommer, and the morifying cold of Winter.

U.   More

Moꝛeouer, their Rootes ſtanding deepe in the ground, they doe the moꝛe eaſily withſtand all eꝛternal iniuries. And when the Spꝛing commeth, and the Sunne ſendeth foꝛth his heate entring into the ſigne of *Aries*, piercing the earth with his quickning beames, hee ſtirreth the ſame, and cauſeth her to open her boſome, out of the which at the laſt ſhee powꝛeth foꝛth abundantly thoſe two liquid beginnings, whereof wee haue ſpoken befoꝛe.

The liquoꝛ, oꝛ Mercurial vapour, which is lifted vp thꝛough the Rootes with Salt Armoniac of a volatile nature (by a certaine wonderfull manner of nature, diſtilling) and aſcending into the trunke, vnder the barke, (at which time trees may eaſily bee diſbarked) raiſeth vp, quickeneth, and adoꝛneth with greene leaues, (trees and plants, now hanging downe their heads, and halfe dead. And the other kinde of volatile ſalt. Nitre-ſulphurus, mixed with the moꝛe volatile ſulphur, and oyle of nature, doth cloath and decke the whole earth euery where with ſundꝛy ſoꝛts of moſt beautiful flowers.

And yet wee muſt not thinke hereupon, that one vapoꝛous liquoꝛ, which pꝛoceedeth out of the earth, is not partaker of the other, ſeeing the Mercurial liquoꝛ is not without his ſulphurus, noꝛ the ſulphurus without his Mercurial. And this is the cauſe why in the vegetable nature, wee doe ſee that ſome doe put out their leaues and flowers ſooner than other ſome.

Nature therefoꝛe hath moſt wiſely diſtributed thoſe beginnings into all things. And experience doth teach, that ſome things doe partake of this oꝛ that, moꝛe than ſome other things. Foꝛ thou canſt not eaſily dꝛaw an oyle out of leaues : but a mercurial liquoꝛ plentifully out of al : and out of very fewe, ſome ſulphurus, oꝛ oylie liquoꝛ The reaſon is, becauſe Mercurie doth carꝛy the rule in leaues, and is their chiefe nouriſhment, beginning and foundatiō as we haue alreadꝛ ſaid. But the ſulphurus liquoꝛ is the cauſe of the increaſe & plentie of flowers, but yet the ſame ſu'phur is not alone and pure, but mixed with ſome poꝛtion of Mercurial liquoꝛ, but with the leaſt quantitie of ſalt.

Mercurie is properly extracted from leaues.

F 03

For this cauſe thou maieſt extract out of flowers, both Sulphur or oyle, and alſo Mercurie, but that oyle more volatil : and
of Salt , the leaſt quantity. But out of ſeedes is extracted
much of the more fixed Sulphur, but of Mercury and Salt
almoſt nothing. The cauſe is , for that Sulphur hath gi- *Sulphur out*
uen beginning and the principal conſtitution, (not that vola- *of Seedes.*
til Nitrous and airey Sulphur, but that which is indeede oyle-
like and fat, and which holdeth a meane betweene fixed and
flying : both which lye hid in ſeedes, euen in thoſe ſeedes which
are in great Mercurial hearbes and fleſhlike fruites, as in Ap-
ples, Peares, Gordes, and ſuch like. But Salt is in all theſe, *Salt out of*
as the moſt fixed and neceſſarie beginning, for the conſtitution *wood and*
and compacting of all bodies. But this Salt doth moſt chiefely *rootes.*
reſide in the wood, and in the roote, not as in his center or proper
ſeate fixed, (for his principal rooting is in the earth) but becauſe
it is firſt and moſt plentifully communicated to the wood and
roote. From hence afterward much is deriued to the branches
and leaues, and but little to the flowers and fruites.

Whereupon out of many leaues a ſufficient quantity of ſalt
may be extracted: but out of flowers and ſeedes a very ſmal quantitie in regard of the others.

Thus you ſee after what maner theſe three beginnings doe
order and determine all vegetables as hypoſtatical beginnings,
and doe bring them forth, conſerue, make them to ſprout and
floriſh, and doe giue vnto them diuers forces and vertues. It is
alſo euident, that the ſaide three beginnings, are in all things, but
in ſome more, and in other ſome leſſe.

Therefore, none of thoſe three beginnings is found ſimple, *A mixture*
and alone, which doth not paticipate alſo with another. For *of the 3. be-*
Salt, through the benefite of the other two Saltes, Niter *ginnings.*
and Armoniac, containeth in it ſelfe an oylely and a Mercuriall ſubſtance : Sulphur containeth a Salte, and a Mercurial ſubſtance : and Mercurie a Sulphurus and Salt ſubſtance.

But euery one of theſe retaineth the name of that, whereof

of it doth moſt partake.

But yet, if we confider of the matter exactly, we ſhal finde
Salt, the root that al the other doe ſpjing from ſalt, as from the firme and con-
of the other ſtant beginning. The nature whereof wil enfoꝛce vs to lift vp
beginnings. our eyes to heauen, ſæing that from theſe interiour and natural
things, that admirable and venerable *Trinitie in Vnitie*, is ſo
clearly and euidently to be ſæne.

And foꝛaſmuch as thoſe thꝛæ ſubſtanceſying beginnings
are, and commonly be found in al the things of nature, wæ muſt
not thinke that they are ſo in them, as without effect, oꝛ vtterly
ſpoiled of al vertue: but wæ muſt rather bæ ſure of the contrarie, namely, that from theſe chiefely, al the qualities, propꝛr-
ties, and vertuals doe ſpꝛing. Foꝛ whatſoeuer hath taſte, the
ſame if it bæ bitter commeth from Salt Gemme. And ſuch
Bitter things haue vertue to clenſe, to euacuate, oꝛ purge. So others
doe purge. which haue in them bitterneſſe, are found to bæ ſuch, as haue
the ſame from this kinde of Salt, and by the benefit thereof, are reckoned among the number of clenſing and purging
medicines. Such are all bitter hearbes, and their Juices. In
like maner all gaules. Foꝛ without theſe thꝛæ, ther can be no due
excretion oꝛ ſeperating in bodies, of ſuperfluities and excrements.
Foꝛ nature by the conduit of her inſtrument, called Choldo-
con, caſting out into the bowels ſome quantitie of gaule, ſtirreth vp the expulſer, and pꝛouoketh it to ſende foꝛth the excrements, and alſo clenſeth, purgeth, and emptieth it ſelfe,
by it ſelfe. The which being vndone, the Expulſer lyeth as it
were buried, and ouerwhelmed, neither is there any good from
thence to be looked foꝛ.

And that bitter Juices, (as alſo the very gaule it ſelfe) are
of the nature of Salt, it may eaſily bee gathered hereby, becauſe
the guale is oftentimes congealed as a fixed Salt into ſtones, in
his owne bladder.

Salt extrac- Alſo out of bitter hearbes, as out of Woꝛme-wood, out
ted out of bit- of the leſſer Centaurie, (which ſome call the gaule of the
ter things. earth) much Salt is extracted, as they that be woꝛkemen know.

Moꝛe-

Hermeticall physicke.

Moreouer out of the gaules of liuing creatures, there is a Salt to bee extracted very bitter, which purgeth wonderfully.
So also there is Salt in vrine, which purgeth the blood by the vaines which send it into the reines, and from thence by the water pipes into the bladder, and so through the conduit thereto Salt in vrine appointed.

In bitter Opium, which all men affirme to be so notably stuperfectiue and cold, there is a bitter and Nitrous Salt, which if thou canst seperate from his stinking Sulphur (by the meanes whereof it is so stuperfectiue) thou shalt make it a notable purger.

So in like maner the skilfull know how to extract out of Centaury, Gentian, Rue, Fumitory, and all such like, very good Purgers. purgers.

Salt which is alluminous, giueth a sower taste: Vitriol a stiptic or a stringent taste: Armoniac a sharpe taste. And a diuers mixture of the same Salts, procureth sundry tastes and relishes: and that most chiefely by the benefit of the two volatile Salts, which of all other wil be best mingled, by reason of their subtilty and spiritous substance. Armoniac, which is sharp, is more plentiful in vitriol, and in things vitriolated, then in any other Salt substance or metallick. For that sharpe Salt, or that sharpenesse of nature, is the fermentation thereof, and the cause of coagulations, and of the dissolutions of all things: as we haue already touched before, and will in another place more manifestly declare. Therefore it is certaine, that those things which are stiptick or stopping, and haue outwardly a greene colour or vitriolated with an inward sharpnesse and certaine redones, (as is to be seene in *Pomegranats*, *Barberies*, and *Limons*) it is certaine that they haue it from vitriol, and from the sharp Salt Armoniac: for the vitriol of nature is outwardly greene, and red within, if thou search it by skilful Anatomie.

So also thou maiest extract out of the barke of the said fruits, as of Granates, a substance comming most neere to the vertue of vitriol. And the liquor which is extracted out of their red graines, Dissoluing liquors. or out of the iuice of *Limons*, or fruite of *Barberies*, hath force to

L 3   dissolue

diſſolue pearles, and coʒall, euen as the ſpirit of bitriol hath. And this commeth by the bertue of Salt Armoniac ſharpe of nature, and by the nature of mixture : but ſo mixed, as by the induſtrie of the artificer it may be ſeperated, in ſuch wiſe, that the ſame Salt Armoniac being extracted, the ſame liquoʒ will be made ſwéete and potable, and the Salt remaine by it ſelfe : the which being againe mixed with ſpʒing water, oʒ with any other liquoʒ denoid of taſte, it wil make the ſame ſharpe.

That ſame ſharpneſſe oʒ Salt Armoniac ſpirituall, is not onely found in Uitriol, but alſo in common Salt, in Niter, yea in Sulphur alſo it ſelfe, as alſo in all things. Foʒ that ſharpneſſe is that very ſame, which coagulateth Sulphur, which is plentifully found therein. Foʒ without it, Sulphur will not cleaue bnited, but would be running, as are other oyle-like liquoʒs.

The ſame Salt Armoniac of nature, is manifeſted bnto bs, by that extraction of ſharpe oyle, which is dʒawen out of Sulphur : whoſe nature is farre different from that of the ſaid Sulphur. Foʒ it is ſo farre from taking ſleame, that contrariwiſe, it is a hinderance to gun-poulder, not ſuffering it to be inflamed with the touch of fire, as is ſaid already. The ſame liquoʒ doth diſſolue pearles and coʒal, no leſſe then doth the iuice of Limons, of Barberies, oʒ any other of that nature, the which power it hath by the diſſoluing bertue of Salt Armoniac of nature which is in it. The like, and by the ſame reaſon, doth Uineger perfoʒme. Foʒ Wine (as is ſaide afoʒe) partaketh of the nature of Uitriol, moʒe then any other begetable, and containeth much of the foʒeſaide ſharpe Salt of nature.

Diſſoluing liquor.

He which doth exactly conſider theſe things, ſhal readily, and out of true grounded reaſons, diſſolue the queſtion, concerning the true and natural qualitie of Uineger, which queſtion hath troubled many of the moſt learned Phyſitians. Foʒ the diſſoluing bertue which appeareth to be in Uineger, euen in this, that when clay oʒ earth is put into it, it wil as it were boyle, argueth that the nature thereof is altogether hote.

Others

Others on the contrary part, denying Uineger to be colde, appoint it as a chiefe remedy to extinguiſh and repreſſe exter nal Inflamations. Alſo by the taſte, which they affirme to bee the effect of colaneſſe, they conclude that Uineger is colde. But they can very eaſily end this controuerſie, which haue the perfect knowledge of the nature of Salt Armoniac, which Uineger containeth in it. For this Salt is the true cauſe of diſſoluing vertue.

But becauſe the ſame Salt is of force to coagulate ſpirits, and to diſſolue bodies, therefore it is effectual, and a ſingular remedy againſt both inward and outward inflamations. For it doth coagulate the Niter Sulphurus exhalations, which ſtirreth vp thoſe inflamations. For ſuch heates and feauerous paſſions, doe proceed out of the ſpirits onely, either Niterous, or Sulphurus, ariſing out of the Salt-Niter Sulphurus or tartarus of our body, and lifted vp into euaporations, which cauſe ſuch vnkindly heates. The which cometh not ſo to paſſe when the ſame ſpirits be as yet bound together, and lye as it they were buried in their proper bodies, or tartarous feces.

But if thou wilt yet knowe more manifeſtly the correſiue force, and inflaming heate of the ſaide ſpirits, conſider the ſtrong waters, (which are nothing elſe but the ſpirits of Niter, and Uitriol) which thou ſhalt ſee will diſſolue ſiluer, or any hard metall. But if thou put but one onely ounce of ſiluer, to one hundred pound waight of Uitriol and Niter, as they are in their owne nature and body, yet they will neuer be able to diſſolue it. *Diſſoluing ſpirits.*

It is therefore manifeſt, that ſuch violent forces and operations, are onely in the ſpirits, ſeperated, euaporated, and diſſolued from their body: the which forces thou ſhalt by no ſafer meanes take away and ſuppreſſe, then if the ſame ſpirits bee againe incorporated, and coagulated. And this is performed by that Salt Armoniac ſharpe of nature, which is in Uineger, as alſo in other things which haue ſharpneſſe.

But peraduenture there are ſome, which now thinking that wee haue killed our ſelues with our owne ſword, will inferre *Obiection.*

feare vpon the fame example by vs alleaged, that fuch eſſences prepared by *Chymiſts*, are all for the moſt part ſpirituall, and therefore by confequence, are moze violent remedies then is fitting

Anſwere.

for nature to beare, and therefoze can not be giuen with ſafetie. J would haue thofe which make this obiection, to be in this wife anfwered. That the reafon is not all one, and therefoze the conclufion not good. Foz if we take the fpirit of Vitriol, oz of Salt-Pæter, which indœd are fpirits partaking of the terreſtriall fire, yet neuertheleſſe they may bee fo ſwœtened, and mingled with bzoathes oz other conuenient liquoz, that they wil be very familiar to nature, grateful, ſauozy, and gentle, and not without great vertue and efficacie. The iuice of *Limons* giuen by it felfe alone into great plenty, can hurt the ſtomack. Foz the which caufe our maner is, to mingle it with fome liquoz, oz with fugar, and to bzing it into a fyzup oz Julep, no leſſe pzofitable then pleaſing to the ſtomach.

The ſpirit of vitriol and his vertue.

But the vertue of the fpirit of vitriol is better knowne at this day, and commended of the moſt appzoued Phyſitians of diuers countries, then that the ignozant can detract any thing from the dignity and pzaife thereof. Jt is repozted very credibly, that in *France* it is much vfed and commented foz the effects it hath to extinguiſh burning feauers. And not without iuſt caufe: foz it is a moſt fingular remedy, not onely againſt feauers, but alfo againſt many other contumacious ſickneſſes, as hereafter in due place, ſhal be ſhewed: but it is fit, that no other pzefume to adminiſter it, then fuch as are expert Phiſitians, not Emperikes, and fuch as try conclufions by killing men.

Furthermoze, the ſharpe fpirit dzawen out of Niter alone, oz Sulphur (among the metallick Salts) is of the fame nature and pzoperty. Foz thefe doe auaile no leſſe then the other, to extinguiſh feauers of what kind foeuer, by their coagulatiue vertue,

A remedy a-gainſt fea-uers.

whereby they doe tame, fubdue, and coagulate, thofe Sulphurs and burning fpirits of our body.

Obiection.

Moreouer, there are other fome, which iudge vs wozthy of much repzehenfion, becaufe we faid afoze, that one and the-felfe-fame ſharpe Salt Armoniac, hath both vertue to diſſolue, and al-

ſ

ſo to congeale: which being effects contrary, cannot proceed from one and the ſame cauſe, according to the common opinion of Phyloſophers.

To this we anſwere, that as we haue ſpoken it, ſo we will maintaine it. And therefore we ſay againe, that this Salt Armoniac ſharpe of nature, whereof we ſpeake, can both diſſolue bodies, and alſo (which is more to be marualled at) congeale ſpirits: yea and which is yet more wonderfull, euen in the middeſt of fire it can congeale.

And concerning diſſolution, it ſhall not be neceſſary that we proue this, becauſe it is well known to perſons of very meane ſkill. And now to ſay ſomewhat for the ignorants ſake: The ſpirit of Uitriol or of Sulphur, or of ſower Niter, wel prepared, and ſeperated from all terreſtreitie, doth diſſolue corall and pearles.

By which diſſolution, an excellent remedy is made to ſtop the fluxes hepatic, *Lienterie*, and *Dyſſenterie*, where the liuer hath need of ſpeedy corroboration. But they muſt neceſſarily be prepared according to Art.

But now time and reaſon perſwadeth vs, that we ſay ſomewhat concerning the contrarie faculty of this ſharpneſſe, which is contrary to the other coagulating effect. To dee this, little wit, and leſſe labour wil ſerue. For they which are but meanely ſeene in the Spargerick Art, and haue bene *Chymiſts* a very ſhort time, or if they be but common Apothecaries, they know this, and haue ſeene it in the preparation of quickſiluer: whoſe liquor and running nature, no exterior coldneſſe, no Elementall froſt, how great ſoeuer the ſame be, congeale or fixe. But if it be ſublimed with Uitriol onely meanely calcined, it will come to paſſe, that Mercury or quick-ſiluer which deſireth his coagulation as his perfection, by a certaine magnetical vertue, draweth into it ſelfe that Sulphur, or that Salt Armoniac ſharpe of nature, by the benefit whereof, of running it is made ſolid and firme, ſo as thou maieſt eaſily handle it.

Being brought into this forme, it is commonly called Sublimate. But to make it yet more perfect, thoſe which are careful and ſkilfull workmen, reiterate their ſublimations, ad-

A remedy to ſtoppe fluxes.

The fixing of quick-ſiluer.

ding

ſing to this new Vitriol, that by his Salt Armoniac of nature, it may be impregnated. And thus at the laſt it becommeth ſolid, and cleare as any Chriſtal Venis-glaſſe.

Spargeric Phyloſophers, can ſo diſpoyle againe this Mercurie ſo prepared, of his coagulation, or of his ſharpe Salt Armoniac of nature, that he ſhal returne to his former ſtate, and offixed ſhal become moueable and running. But he is now perfectly clenſed, and is now no more common Mercury or Hydrargyre, but the Phyloſophers Mercury.

Mercurie of the Phyloſopher.

And now, if the foreſaid water be exhaled or vapozed, that there may remaine nothing but a ſharpe liquoz, like vnto the ſpirit of Vitriol, thou ſhalt haue a liquoz moze excellent then any Vitriolated ſpirit, and truly ſpirituall. And ſo in ſtæde of a great poyſon which was mixed with Mercurie (which was then nothing but a certaine terreſtrial corroſiue fire) thou ſhalt now haue the true ſpirit of Vitriol: whoſe greater and better part vapozeth away, is conſumed and loſt, if it bee extracted accozding to the common manner, with that great and violent fire by Retozt.

The right ſpirit of Vitriol good againſt the falling euil.

This ſpirit prepared after the ſaide manner, is excæding good, and a ſpecial commaunder of the Epilepſie, if it be adminiſtred by a ſkilful Phyſitian, not by an Emperick, with proper and conuenient liquoz. And this is one tryal of the vertue of coagulating Mercury.

The ſame coagulating force of his doth manifeſtly appeare in thoſe prepalations which are called precipitations, which are made with the ſharpe ſpirits of Vitriol and of Sulphur, by the meanes whereof it may be brought into a poulder, which cannot be eaſily done by fire.

A remedy for Gangrena, & eating vlſers.

But that it may appeare that this coagulating power of Armoniac of nature, is not onely vppon Mercurie, (ouer whome it can exerciſe this power) but nothing at all vpon the ſpirits Niter-Sulphurus of our bodies, with the which quickſiluer hath no ſimpathy, oz conuenience) we wil ſhew it by a certaine other manifeſt demonſtration, and the ſame moſt true: as ſhall appeare to them which will try it. And in the ſame experiment

Hermeticall Physicke.

experiment I wil also teach a very excellent remedy against Gangrena, and all sorts of cankerous Ulcers : if any bee loth to take it inwardly into the body, because of the vrine ingredient.

Take the vrine of a boy, betwæne the age of ten and sixtæne, which drinketh wine in good quantity: let it be depured according to Art : Adde hereunto of *Romane*, or *Hungarian* Uitriol (for by these the operation wil be the better) I say of the Uitriol, twise so much. Put it to digestion in Balneo Mar, which is moyst, by the space of sire or eight dayes, in one, or in seuerall glasse Allembicks. For there is required much matter. This digestion being ended, thou shalt increase the fire of Balne til the water sæthe. Presently set on a head with a receiuer, and distill the water.

And the same which first commeth forth, is an excellent Ophthalmick water for the eyes. The second something more sharp then the former, is excellent good to asswage the paines of the Gout.

Thus goe forward, vrging the heate of the Balne, or else by hote asshes, vntill the matter in the bottom of the Alembic remains like vnto hony. The which afterward thou shalt put into an yron vessel, and putting fire vnder it, stirre it continually with an yron spattle, that it cleaue not too : this thou shalt continue so long, vntill all the liquor is vapored away, and that there remaineth onely the Salt of Uitriol, and of the vrine dry in the bottome, and in a certaine masse. This being pouldred, put it into a cornute, wel luted, hauing a wide receiuer, wel closed, that the spirits issue not forth. Then put to a vehement fire, (such as is nædful for the making of strong water, or the spirit of Uitrioll.

But the fire must bee moderated by degrées, vntill it come to the highest degrée, as Art requireth . And then at the last you shall sæ the receiuer filled euery where with white spirits, which in that great heate will be congealed as it were into Ise-sickels, hauing all bout the body of the receiuer:

Water for the Ophthalmie.

Water to ease the gout.

✳ 2　　　　　　much

much like onto the hayfe oz white thzedes, which in time of froſt are congealed out of foggy miſtes, and doe hang vpon the trees. Thefe are the fpirits of the Salt, which through the vehement heate of the fire, are thus fozmed.

A remedy a-
gainſt obſer-
uations, and
to breake the
Stone.

This Iſe may be kept, after the maner of Salt Piter. Wherof if thou giue one fcruple oz halfe a fcruple, in bzoath, wine, oz other conuenient liquoz, it will ſhewe it felfe an excellent remedy againſt all obſtructions of the Liuer and of the fpleene, it pzouoketh vzines, and is alfo a fpecial remedy againſt the Stone.

Gangrena
cured.

The fame Iſe being bzought into water (foz it will eafily be diſſolued) is a pzincipal remedy foz Inflamations and Gangrenas, which very fodainly it extinguiſheth. Out of this fo faire and noble experient, euery true Phylofopher and Phyſitian,

Caufes of the
Stone.

will take occaſion of feeking and fearching further then the common fozt are woont: and fo he may moze certainly finde out the caufes of ſtones congealed, which are ingendzed of thefame falts oz tartarous matter in diuers parts of our body.

He will alfo haue moze quick infight into many other difeafes which come by the coagulation of the fozefaid ſharp and Vitriolated fpirits, oz elfe of the euapozations of other moſt ſharpe fpirits, from whence Inflamations, and gouty paines with fwellings doe fpzing, by the inward vertue of the thickened fpirits afozefaid. Thefe things being thus knowne, a remedy wil eafily be found to mittigate, and to diſſolue fuch calculous and ſtony matter, if we marke and confider diligently, where that ſharpe vertue lyeth hidden, and wherein alfo the coagulatiue pzopertie of the faid fpirits are.

Alfo the fame contemplation, will giue occafion to pzie into the diuers and fundzy meteozs, which ſhewe themfelues in man, the little wozld, out of thofe continual vapours and exhalations which are lifted vp from the lower belly (which we fitly cōpare with the earth) into the aire, that is to fay, into the vppermoſt region of the body, the bzaine. So it ſhal appeare, that from the Mercurial vapours, thickened into cloudes through the coldneſſe of the bzaine, and by the fame not able to be difpzeſſed, doe fall fometimes moderate ſhowers, and fimple in ſhewe,

and

and fometime out of thicke clouds abundance of waters. Wherof come either gentle Rheumes, o; violent catarres, which are
called fuffocatiue, becaufe the matter ruſheth after a certaine violent maner, vpon the vital partes. Furthermore, out of the fame
contemplations thou ſhalt finde the true o;iginal of windes, of
haile, of ſnowe, whereof commeth the tingling in the eares, the
Palfey, the Apoplexe, and ſuch like defeafes, ſtirred vp from the
Mercurial thickened vapours. The which difeafes come not (as
fome doth thinke) becaufe of coloneſſe onely : but the caufe alfo
thereof is the ſharpeneſſe of Salt vitriolated, which being mixed
with thofe Mercurial vapours, doth fuddenly coagulate and congeale them: and this is the caufe of Apoplexes and ſuch like. For
to take an example from our owne body, to manifeſt this thing,
the v;ine which we make, is fo repleniſhed with thefe mercurial
humours, mixed with ſharpe falt, that it hath fo;ce and power to
coagulate. Wherefo;e this which wee haue faide muſt ſimply
be granted vnto vs that Salt Armeniac of natural ſharpe, hath *Sal-Armo-*
fo;ce to diſſolue bodies, and to coagulate fpirits, as wee haue *niac a coagu-*
plainely declared in the fo;efaid experiments. *lator and a*
diſſoluer.

But paraduenture fo:ne yong fcoffing Scholler, which neuer knew what Phylofophie ment, with great confidence and
no ſhame (as of late one which ſhewed him felfe an Aſſe and a
Calfe, and yet of a ripe wit did) dare rife vp againſt vs and fay,
that in our body, no vitriolated nature can bæ found, no; any
thing like vnto it. But this fellowe and fuch like, wee wil
teach fufficiently and moderately (if they wil not refufe to learne)
in our boke concerning the hidden nature of things, and the perfection of art, where wee wil declare this thing, and many other
p;ofitable queſtions, neceſſary fo; a true Phiſitiar. But yet not
to let the matter vtterly paſſe, without fome thing fpoken concerning this point, I wil vtter my felfe in fewe wo;ds.

Firſt of al I wiſh, that exact confideration bæ had, which is
that fire of nature, and which is the authour of the concoction of
meate in our ſtomach, which diſſolueth ϝchaungeth the fame, and
that in fo ſho;t a time, as neither ſæthing water, no; elementarie

fire can doe, no not in long time. Let them alfo I pray you confider what is the caufe of that dog-like appetite which fome men
haue, by which they are wont fo readily to confume all the meat
in their ftomach, that nature hath fcarce lawful fpace to nourifh
her felfe: and from whence this infatiable hunger commeth.
Accoding to the common opinion, it befalleth fome man to haue
this appetite, by reafon of a certaine fharpe and melancholick humour, which being thruft downe into his fides, doth fometimes
boyle vp like moft ftrong vinegar, or rather in deed like oile of vi-

The caufe of dogge-like appetite.
triol, or like fome fuch diffoluing and deuouring thing. For truly, if that fharpneffe were diligently confidered, and thoughly
looked into by Phylofophical anatomie, it would eafily be iudged
by good and indifferent men, that it fhould not moe vnfitly to
bee fayde vitriolated, than melancholicke: nay moe aptly and
better: becaufe melancholie, neither can, no hath been wont
to woke fuch effects, except by the fowreneffe aforefaid. For
by this manner of fpeaking, the diffoluing vertue, and al other
properties, are in farre better fot expreffed, which fhal eafily
appeare in him which wil thoughly fcanne and weigh al
things.

And what doth let vs now, fo call fuch faculties and humours
vitriolated, when as al their properties and forces, doe come fo
neere to the nature of vitriol? Shal it bee free and permitted to

**Choller, ru-
ftie, yeallow, and greene.**
common Phyfitians, to cal choler, *Æruginus, Vitelline, & Pro-
racious*, for the likeneffe & affinitie of thofe things from whence
the name is borrowed: and why then fhal it not bee lawful for
vs to doe the like, and to fay that humors are vitriolated, becaufe they partake of the nature of vitriole?

But let vs returne to our Meteors which are in our bodie:
hauing already fpoken of them which are raifed vp by the vapours of mercurial liquors, which haue a fimilitude with the watery, and alfo with thofe which proceed out of the meere vapours
of the earth of the great world. Now it remaineth that wee fay
fomething alfo of the others.

Therefore euen as as the vapours and exhalations fulphurus, Nitrous, or Antimonial, carryed vp out of the earth into the

Ayre

Hermeticall Phyſicke.

Ayre and cloudes, doe cauſe fiery Meteors, Corruſcations, Lightnings, Thundrings, Comets, and ſuch like: euen ſo alſo in our
bodyes, from the fumes and ſmoakie euapozations procæding
from burnt and ſcozched blood, and from ſo manifold and diuers
tartarous, ſulphurus, and niterous fumes, with the which our
bowels doe abound, the like Meteors are produced. Foz ſuch
fuming matter, lying burning in the ſides, nære to the Liuer
and the Sploene, hindered by windineſſe, being thereof cauſed,
oz elſe ſtirred vp by an immoderate and feauerous heate, being
at the the laſt lifted vp and carried into the bzaine, and therin ſet
on fire, ſtirre vp Meteors, long madneſſes, burning phzenzies,
ſetled melancholies, dotings, paines of the head, falling ſickneſſes, and many ſuch like. Some of theſe continue long, by reaſon of the clammie hardineſſe oz abundance of the matter, as
madneſſe: other ſome are ſoner gone, as Phzenſies: ſome doe
moze fearſely exerciſe a man, ſome moze gently, accozding as
the ſaide fuming matters bæ moze oz leſſe ſharpe, abundant,
cleauing, Salt, ſulphurus, oz of qualitie moze oz leſſe inflame-
able, oz by any manner of other meanes hurtfull. Foz there
is great diuerſitie of theſe fumie matters: no leſſe than wæ
ſæ differences of fires and ſmeakes in combuſtible woods,
whereof ſome are moze clammie, ſome moze ſalt, ſome ſulphurus, and ſuch like diuerſities.

The ſame diuerſitie alſo is to bæ ſæne in the ſeparation of
the ſpirits of Léeſe, of Ale, of Cider, of Wine, of *Hydromel*,
and of ſuch like dzinkes, the diuerſitie whereof doth manifeſtly
appeare, by the odours which doe abundantly aſcend into the
noſe.

Alſo in Saltes, Sulphurs and oyles, which are diſtilled, the
diuerſitie of vapoures, (which are nothing but the ſpirits pzo-
duced out of many tartarous matters) doe manifeſtly declare the ſame. Foz of theſe, ſome are ſharpe, ſome ſowze,
ſome biting, ſome ſtinking, ſome odoziferous, ſome ſo
pearcing, that the very odour doth ſtrike the bzayne, and
doe cauſe extraozdinary neſſing, oz elſe by ſome other
meanes

*The Philo-
ſophical
cauſe of
Meteors
&c.*

*The cauſe of
madneſſe,
Phrenſie,
and ſuch
like.*

meanes doe hurt the braine, dazeling, dulling, or troubling the
ſpirits, or elſe by fumes which are ſulphurus and ſtupefactiue.

The ſame differences are to be made in Antimonials, Arſenicals, and Mineral humours, or vapours, and that out of their
effect, either ſeptic putrifying, or cauſtic burning, the which effects
are in the ſaid fumes, by the meanes of ſalt. Such pearcing
fumes are too wel knowne, and felt of our eyes oftentimes, to
which they bring by their ſharpeneſſe, paines, inflamations, and
flowing of teares. Hereupon out of this diuerſitie of fumes,
there ariſe diuers paſſions, in continuance, in maladie, and in ve-
niencie, more or leſſe inuading and troubling, according to the
nature, mineral, and condition of the qualitie or quantitie of the
erhalations, and of their ſubſtances, which are lifted vp with
them, as it were in a certaine chariot.

Moreouer, we ſee in the bowels of the earth of the little world,
man, no leſſe then in the great worlds belly : in the bellies I ſay
of both, almoſt the ſame effects are to bee ſeene of Meteors, as
wel waterie as fierie. For example, the Tympanie, the ſwelling
of the Coddes, windineſſe of the ſtomach, and bellie : al which
doe repreſent the windes, raynes, and Earth-quakes of the
earth : and the waters within the body, and betweene the ſkin
and the fleſh, doe repreſent the Sea, the Riuers and Springs of
the earth.

Alſo there are in man diuers fierie Meteors, by reaſon of
the erhalations, of the Niterous and Sulphurus ſpirits, which
being ſet on fire, ſtirre vp ſuch diuerſities of Feauers and inflamations.

There are bred alſo in man, diuers metallic ſubſtances, as
ſandes, and ſtones, which are commonly ingendered in diuers
parts of his bodie, as in his bowels, ſtomach, gaule, ſplæne, lyuer, yea, in the lunges and braine : but more often in the reynes
and bladder, which are the moſt fertile mines of al the reſt.

There are alſo procreated in mans bodie, certaine concreate &
congealed Juices; as many kindes of Sulphurs, but of Saltes
more differences, vitriolated, alluminous, niterous, and Gem-
mous. Salt-gemmie, or common ſalt, is plentifull in Salt ſpittle.

ſower Salt-Armoniac, in ſower flegme oʒ ſpittle, and alſo in a
certaine kinde of ſower melancholy: ſalt vitriolated and of the
colour of ruſtie metal, in choller that is of the ſame complexion:
Salt aluminous, pʒicking and ſtipticke, in glaſſy fleame, of the
ſame qualitie: Salt nitrous and bitter, in bitter choller. Moʒe-
ouer, Vʒines which are wholy niterous, due repʒeſent a matter
moſt like to Niter. There are alſo in this little woʒlde, as alſo
in the greater woʒld, found many differences of Salts: as a ſu-
gered ſalt, in ſweete flegme: as alſo an Arſenical and coʒroding
Salt, in malignant and peſtilent humours. Fʒom the reſoluti-
ons of the which Saltes, but moſt eſpecially of the ſtiplick oʒ coʒroding ſalts, come certaine kindes of Chollickes, which afterwards degenerate into contractions of the bowels: Fʒom
the coʒroſiue Salts ſpʒing diuers kindes of diſenterie fluxes:
from the bʒiniſh ſalts, come the burnings of Vʒines: from the
tart Salts, commeth the appetite of the Stomach: from the
Arſenicall Salts, comes Carbuncles, cankerous Vlcers, runing
pockes, & ſuch like. And of the congelations of theſe ſalts, comes
Goutes, Stones, Scirrhus hardneſſe, and diuers kindes of obſtructions, accoʒding to the diuerſitie of tartars, and of Salts
which are ingendʒed and pʒocreate to nature, in our body. Fʒom
theſe things, are the cauſes of diſeaſes in mans body, to be truely
and exactly learned and diſcerned: without the which wæ ſhal in
vaine ſæke foʒ remedies.

Salts of di-
uers kinds in
mands body.

But to make al which, hath bæene hitherto ſpoken moʒe plaine,
wæ wil adde certayne manifeſt demonſtrations, and plague
to ſenſe, but yet in as bʒiefe manner as I can, ſæing wæ haue
reſerued a moʒe ample and ſpecial Treatiſe of theſe things to our
woʒke, concerning the hidden nature of things.

It is known and confeſſed of al, by the Edict of *Hyppocrates*,
the chiefeſt Authour of Phiſitians, that our body conſiſteth of
things containing of things contained, and of things en-
foʒcing. The things containing, are the ſolide and moʒe firme
partes, as the bones, griſtles, ligaments, fleſh, which doe
containe, and as it were reſtraine, the moʒe ſoft and delicate
parts.

P   The

The contents are in a two fold difference: ſome are violen-
breathing out, and enforcing: (as Phyſitians ſpeake) other-
ſome moyſtening, and flowing out. The firſt ſort, are the ſpirits of our radical Balſam, which they call naturall ſpirits,
whether they be firmely fixed in any one part, or whether
they haue ſcope and recourſe throughout the whole body; generated of the moſt pure ſubſtance ſpiritual of the Sulphurus liquor, and of the ſalts of the nouriſhments of our life. Furthermore, they diuide the ſpirits, into natural, vital, and animal.

All theſe, are either natural and pure, or elſe impure and feculent. The one are of a moſt pure nature, ethereal and conſer-
uers of life: the other groſſe and impure in compariſon of them,
ſubiect to alterations; for that they participate much of the feculent impuritis of Mercurie, and of the liquors of Salt, and alſo
of the aliments of Sulphur: of the which beginnings wee doe
conſiſt, as wee ſaid before. The moyſtening parts are mercurial liquors, or that which they commonly call humours, as
well the natural, profiting and nouriſhing, which retaine ſomewhat of the ſpirit of life, as the vnprofitable and excremental.

The out-flowing and breathing forth, are the breathes, vnder
which name alſo wee comprehend the vapours, of the which we
made mention before: which vapours are a diſtillation, and that
moyſt euapozation, taken from the more watery part of humo-
ral or mercurial things: or elſe a dry exhalation, of Sulphurus
and tartarous things, and of Salts of our body.

And ſuch exhalations alſo are no other thing, but fumes and
ſpirituall ſmoakes, but yet excremental, and therefore ſuperfluous. For beſide thoſe firſt ſeperations, which nature maketh
out of the more groſſe part of nouriſhments, by the excretion
and ſeparation of the ordinarie impure feces: there are yet alſo in the *Chylus*, or good Iuice, and in the very blood,
which of all other humours are moſt noble, certaine ſuperfluous impurities, which for the ſame cauſe Nature ſeperateth.

Therefore the more moyſt ſuperfluities are ſeparated by euapozations, and thoſe onely which are ſeperated in the third concoction.

coction, which could not be made ſemblable o2 like to the nouriſhing parts. Fo2 the which cauſe nature expelleth them by inſenſible paſſages, euē th2ough the po2es of the ſkin, that our natural heate may the mo2e freely be winded by the ay2e, and the burning of the heart comfo2ted.

The b2eathing ſuperfluities alſo, doe paticipate as much of
the d2ie as of the moyſt: that is to ſay, of thoſe which are exhaled
and euapo2ated out of the ſulphurus ſalt matters, and mercurial
liquo2s. Whereof the mo2e thinne and b2eathie part, paſſe by
inſenſible tranſpirations: the mo2e waterie, by ſweates: but
the mo2e foule, and that which is feculent, cleaueth to the out-
ſide of the ſkinne.

But now, if ſuch vapouring exhalations be retained ſtil in our
body, (the which ſometime commeth to paſſe th2ough the cold-
neſſe of the ay2e cōpaſſing vs about, by the ſh2inking of the ſkin, *The ſtopping*
by occaſion of place, o2 of age, by intemperate life, by a naturall *of the pores*
diſpoſition, by the thickneſſe of the ſkinne, o2 by ſuch like occaſi- *procureth*
ons) then it cannot be, but that ſuch bodies ſhal be ſubiect to ma- *ſickneſſe.*
ny other diſeaſes, than thoſe whereof we haue ſpoken befo2e.

It is alſo to bee rememb2ed in this place, that in all theſe eua-
po2ations, & o2dinarie exhalations, ſomewhat of our ſubſtance-
ſp2ing nectar of life, o2 of our radical Balſam, doth alſo b2eathe a-
way. The which b2eathing, if it be gently and ſparingly, and
without all manner violence and fo2ce, but by a certaine volun-
tarie continuance, and naturall, then our age is p2olonged, in the
meane time declining to extreame old age by little and little, vntill al our water of life, o2 radical oyle (which continueth the
lampe of our life) be conſumed.

But if the ſayd exhalation o2 b2eathing bee violently
and ſuddenly enfo2ced, as it commeth to paſſe in burning ſea-
ſons, and in many other ſickneſſes, faintings, paſſions, and
moſt vehement motions of the ſpirits of our body then our life
ſhall be p2euented befo2e age. Heereupon commeth the vntimely, and in ſome ſo2t, the violent death of many: and yet the cauſe
of ſuch violence comming from an internal occaſion.

And

And becaufe it is very pertinent and neceffarie, that wée rightly vnderftand thofe things which wée haue now fpoken, concerning the natures of the contents in vs , that is to fay, of the enforcings , morftenings, and out-flowings ? and fo much the rather,becaufe by them wée come to the knowledge of our fpirits, and of our radicial moyfture, oz nectar of life, and alfo to the caufes of the conferuation, prolongation, deftruction, and abzeuiation of our life, I wil therefoze now declare them all by an example , whereby euery one which wil giue eare, may come to the perfect knowledge of thofe things.

And yet wée doe not much eftéeme prefumptions, probable reafons, oz authozities, but wée wil ground our demonftration vppon the very fenfes themfelues, that thofe things which wée fpeake , may bée both féene and felt. And if fo bée any bée fo farre deuoyd of fhame,that hée will yet obftinately contradict vs, we will fay to him, as fometime *Auerrho* faid : *One experience is more of value,than many reafons.* Experience cannot bée without fenfe: he which denieth fenfe,is worthy to haue no vfe of fenfe.

And forafmuch as *Ariftotle* fayd, that the foundation of all demonftration is in fenfe, Who is hée that dare gainefay it ?

Therefoze wée wil take Wine againe foz an example, forfomuch as wée vfed the fame befoze. In which wine how apparantly and manifeftly doe fuch feparations , and excrements appeare to bée made ? And this it doth by his owne proper nature, that the moze eafily the nature of either of them, and of both, may manifeftly bée knowen by this Analogie and refemblance which it hath with our blood. Foz by the clenfing of wine , wée know the vitall Anatomie of our blood : and by the fame it will appeare which are our natural fpirits ethereal,as alfo which is our natiue heate, and radicall moyfture, which two doe vphold our body , and defend our life, and of whofe helpe either of them haue néede: forafmuch as that radicall moyfture is the foode and nourifher of heate, and this fame heate fubfifteth by the benefite of that moyfture.

Thus

Thus theſe two repleniſhed with ſpirit, and as it were knit together, are ſpred and diffuſed through the whole body. By this ſame example, the difference betwéene nouriſhing vital humiditie, and that which is vnprofitable and excremental, wil plainly appeare. Furthermore, it wil appeare which be moyſt, and which be dry, in that kind of moyſtures which are outflowing : and which of them are hurtful to our nature, and which profitable. By which anatomie of blood, the reader willing to learne, ſhal profit more (as I thinke) becauſe we referre thoſe foure humors, (whereof they make blood one) to the very ſame, and doe by a certaine analogie and reſemblance, compare it therewith But to come to the matter.

Therefore when the wine is prepared, the cluſters of grapes are cruſhed in the wine-preſſe firſt, and the ſkinnes and kernels with the ſtalkes are throwne away. Then the vnprofitable clenſings and excrements, being partly by mans induſtrie, and partly by the nature of the wine it ſelfe being reiected, the wine is powred into calkes and veſſels. In theſe, digeſtion being made, by his owne force, it ſeperateth and purgeth forth together thoſe feculent and more groſſe ſuperfluities. This done, the wine is all moſt perfect, and fit for drinke and nouriſhment.

That firſt artificiall preperation of wine, (which is made by the expreſſion and ſeparation of the Wintners) doth after a certaine manner repreſent vnto vs, the preparation of wheate, in the which ſeparation, the chaffe and the branne being taken away, the reſt is ground into meale, that it may be more fit for nouriſhment. Even ſo in like maner in our mouthes firſt preparation of the fleſh is made from the bones, or ſuch like : And the expreſſion or grinding is made with the mouth and téeth, then after due chewing, the meate is ſent downe into the ſtomach. This is the firſt reſembled preparation of our nouriſhment, with that firſt preparation of wine, and wheate, and that which is put into our ſtomach, anſwereth that wine, which at the firſt is put into veſſels, & the meale which is ground. Therefore after this, there is another working in the ſtomach by nature. For whatſoeuer the ſtomach receiueth, it concocteth, and digeſteth: yea all kind of

meates

meates mixed together, like wine in his caske, or any other kind of drinke, made of hony, fruites, barley, or of water wherein diuers things are sodden.

The stomach therefore is that vessell of nature, wherein not only the matter put into it is concocted and digested: but also it is the same which seperateth the tartarous feces, and whatsoeuer is excremental therein, by such passages and vents, as nature hath prouided to that end. At the length after much purifying, the blood is clensed, being the red fountaine, and the originall of the spirits of our life: euen like as wine which throughly fined is preferred before all others, which serue for the nourishing and restoring of our life. But let vs now procede.

Out of this artificiall wine, with the helpe of gentle fire, by circulatorie vessels (as they terme them) is extracted a fire of nature, which attendeth the radicall moysture: namely, a water of life, wholy fiery and ethereal, a quintessence, altogether spirituall, and almost of an incorruptible nature.

After the very same manner, through the benefite of nature, and by Circulation which is made by the heate of the Heart, and of the Liuer, there is generated and extracted in vs that quickening fire, accompanied and nourished with his proper vnctuous humour, and radicall, which is the water of life, and true and quickening Nectar, the quint sence, and almost the ethereall spirit, the incorruptible vpholder and conseruer of our life.

This also here by the way commeth to be noted in the operatiõ of the foresaid wine, which is also worthy the marking and admiration: namely, that two or three fiery coales and no moe, *Spirit of wine.* put vnder a large vessel or chaldron, (which may containe fixe gallons, will heate the same wine, and will procure the spirit of wine to distill: when as by that small heate, a much lesse portion of water, cannot bee made blood warme. But which is more to bee maruailed at and obserued, when the same spirit of wine, doth passe through the Colunrina (as they terme it) namely by very long conduites and pipes of brasse retorted, fit for this distillation, it doth so heate them, as also a whole pipefull pipeful of cold water beſide, and farre enough from fire, (in the which the ſaide pipes are moyſtened) that a man may ſcarce handle them. The which is to bee attributed to the great heate which the ſpirit of wine giueth to the colde water paſſing through the foreſaide pipes. For when all the ſpirit of wine is diſtilled forth, although thou put vnder the ſaide veſſell a much more vehement fire, yet thou ſhalt feele the heate of that water in the veſſel contained, to bee extinguiſhed and cooled. The which ſhould put vs in minde what is the next cauſe and originall of natural or connatural heate in vs: for this heate is ſtirred vp in vs by the continual circulation of the quickening ſpirit of our blood.

When all this water of life is at laſt diſtilled forth by a certaine internal, external, and violent heate, or elſe vtterly waſted by progreſſe of time, then doth appeare the extinction of that quickening heate, and cold death inſueth. But to returne to the matter.

After the extraction of the true *Aqua-Vitæ*, or ſpirit of wine, (which is the whole purity of thoſe three ſubſtantial beginnings) whoſe liquor repreſenteth Mercury, whoſe flame, which it readily conceiueth, ſheweth the Sulphurus nature, and the exceeding ſtrong taſte, declareth the ſpirit of Salt Armoniac) there remaineth great plenty of ſteame, or of Mercurial water, which as yet containeth ſome quantity of ſpirit of wine.

But the laſt remainder is no better then vnprofitable water, which ſoone corrupteth in like manner, after the extraction of the water of life, (which is truly ſpiritual,) from out of our blood, there remaineth in our body, that moyſt and moyſtening liquor, which is partly nouriſhing, and partly excrementall, as is ſaide afore. Laſtly, there remaine ouer and aboue the former, the Feces Tartarous reſidences, and Piterus Sulphurus matter, which containe many ſtinking Impurities, as alſo greate plentie of Salt.

The impurities, vox ſufficiently ſhewes the impurities in

the

the eyes, and filthy ftinkes out of the nofthzrils, where as diuers oyles are diftilled out of the faid feces by vehement fire. And out of the very feces there is extracted Salt, if they be calcined, and the fame is alfo fired with his pzoper fteame, as we haue fhewed afoze in the wozking of the fame vegetable. This Salt is made Uolatil, with Salt Armoniac, flying contained in his own fpirit, oz water of life, pzocæding as we haue already fhewed.

In like fozt in blod, befide that fpirit of life and Mercurial liquoz, (which two may in very dæde be feperated from blod it felfe, and fhewed to the eye, after conuenient digeftions, in the heate of *Balne Mary*, which refembleth the heate of nature, that it may the better and moze eafily appeare, how the fame heate, and the fame nature in vs, maketh the fame feperations and operations) J fay, befide thofe two, a certaine foft confiftence like liquoz, wil refide in the bottome, wherein thou fhalt finde many impurities, to be fæns and fmelt, if the fame matter be dzyed vpon a fire of afhes, pzopoztionable to the heate of a feauer, and no greater.

This Alter-Sulphurus ftinke is that, which manifeftly caufeth in vs fiery meteozs, as wel in the vpper, as in the inferiour part of the body, and which bzingeth fozth innumerable paffions and paines befide, as is already fhewed afoze.

So alfo by the fozce of the fire, Sulphurs and oyles, thick and gluing like pitch, may be feperated out of the feces and tartar of blod, no leffe then out of wine, fo offenfiue with ftinke, as thou art not able to abide the odour thereof: whereof, how many difeafes may arife in our bodies, euery man may eafily coniecture

This done, there wil remaine afhes, out of which a Salt is extracted, the which (by the vertue of the Salt Armoniac of nature) may be made Uolatil, and the very fame which *Lullie* calleth the greater *Lunarie*, foz the imitation of the vegetable wozk. This wozke is very admirable, by which the true Mumie, the vniuerfal Medicine, and the true Balfam conferuing and reftoring nature is made. And this is the true and vital anatomie of blod, which by manifeft demonftration we haue fhewed, that it hath a great analogie, pzopoztion and refemblance with wine: when

when as a true Phyloſopher, as wel out of the one as out of the other (ſauing that the one requireth greater artifice) knoweth how to ſeperate waters of life meerely ſpirituall, which are ſaide to be very forcible and ſtrong : and beſide theſe, Mercuriall liquors, which are as wel profitable as hurtfull, which are alſo moyſtening: and finally, which knoweth how to extract vapors, and exhalations fuming, which are called out-flowings.

Now therefore, if ſo be in wine, which we eaſily vſe to nouriſh our bodies, and the ſame pure and cleare after the ſeperation of the ſpirit thereof, we ſee and behold ſo many vnkindly things, and ſo impure ; how many more groſſe impurities I pray you ſhall we finde in the Lées of wines cleauing to the caſkes, and in the groſſe reſidence of the ſame ?

They which knowe and vnderſtand that great and exceeding blackneſſe of wine lées (which is manifeſtly to be ſéene in the calcination thereof) and the ſepreation of his ſpirit, and of his oyle, red, blacke and ſtinking, which is done by deſtillation, they (I ſay) can giue cleare teſtimony and credibly informe, what a great ſtinke there is in the Sulphur thereof : and how great the acrimony and byting ſharpneſſe is in the ſame tartar or lées, by reaſon of the Salt which is extracted out of the ſame, and the oyle which is made by the reſolution of the ſame Salt of tartar. And truſt mée, in the feces of the ſame wine, there are found, beſide the things already ſpoken, thoſe matters which are more groſſe, impure and ſtinking, as they wel knowe, who to calcine them into aſhes (which they call clanelated) are compelled to goe out of the Cities into the fieldes, and places further off by reaſon of their exceeding infection and ſtinke, with the which they are wont to infect the places néere adioyning.

What maruaile is it then, as is ſhewed afore, if in our blood, after the ſeperation of the true ſpirit, there are found ſo many vnkindly, tartarous, ſtinking and Sulphurus impurities ? But what maruaile I ſay, if more and greater impurities and ſtinkes, are to bee found in diuers of the Heterogeneal parts of the Chylus, or beſt matter digeſted in the

Z   Stomach

ftomach fo2 nourifhment, from whence blood d2aweth his firft beginning of his compofition? That tartar o2 lées, is of the blood
which cleaueth to the veffels of the bowels . Now the feces of
the Chylus are nothing elfe, but that huge heape of excrements
of diuers fo2ts, which are in that nourifhment exifting in diuers
parts of the body. And when thofe Niter-Sulphurus and tartarous impurities, cannot by nature be digefted, ouercome and
expelled, they ftuffe the bowels, they are made the feminarie and
fto2e-houfe of moft grieuous ficknettes : fo that if we will con-
fette ǧ truth, we muft of neceffity fay with great *Hipocrates*, that
ficknettes haue both their féedes, and alfo their roles in our bo-
dies:the which moft euidently appeareth by the fo2efaide comparifon of wine and blood. The which ftandeth vpon apparant
and fenfible foundations, and not vpon doubtfull figments and
Imaginations.

And as we fée in the fp2ing times, when nature putteth fo2th
her flowers, that the lées of wine, are mixed with the wine it
felfe, and doe trouble it, and oftentimes co2rupt it : and that
as in the excéeding heate of the Sommer Sunne, the mo2e hote
Sulphurus part of the fame wine, that is, the fpirit, may and
is wont to vapour away, whereof followeth the co2ruption
of the fame wine:euen fo alfo, about the fame feafons and times,
the feces, and tartarous heape mixed with our blood, doth at
the laft peruert, and co2rupt it: hereof commeth the occafion
and multiplication of ficknettes. Fo2 the fpirit of blood being
difp2earced and feperated, both by external and alfo by internal heate, it muft nédes bé co2rupted, to the which co2rup-
tion, arifing of the faid caufes, the caufe of many ficknettes is
rather to be referred, then to thofe bare fimple qualities, of hote
and cold, d2y and moyft.

As therefo2e we haue taught in the feperation of the true fpirit of wine (which refembleth the celeftiall and fpiritual Nectar
of our life) many impurities thereof doe manifeftly appeare:euen
fo, and after the very fame fo2t, it fareth with wheate with fruits,
and with meates and d2inkes p2epared of them , and generally
with all other vegetable things, p2océeding after the fame maner
as

as we haue ſaid,concerning wine. For they haue no light proportion with our bloud,accoding to this ſaying: We are nouriſhed
with thoſe things whereof we conſiſt : which thou maieſt aptly
turne and ſay; we conſiſt of thoſe things, wherewith we are nouriſhed . But the one partaketh of the other, oz of this oz of that
moze then of the other : as foz example, of the ſpirit, of the Mercuriall liquoz, of Salt, of the feces, & of the ſtinking & vnprofitable
excremēts: which is the reaſon, that out of this oz that moze commendable kinde of meate, the moze wozthy and commendable
bloud is generated.

Therefoze to adde one example moze in ſtéed of a ſurpluſſage
of waight, let it not be fozgotten , that out of Hydzomel, Cider,
Ale, oz ſuch like kind of dzinkes, & out of their feces, the ſame preparations and ſeperations, as wel of a commendable liquoz, as
of feces, may be made after the ſame maner, as we haue befoze
ſhewed to be done concerning wine : and that the beginnings
and heterogeneall and vnnaturall parts, may in the ſame ſozt be
extracted out of theſe, as out of that other.

To conclude, thou maieſt with better ſucceſſe learne the beginnings of ſickneſſes , by making a compariſon betwéene the
preparation and ſeperation of thoſe things which giue nouriſhment vnto man, and our bloud, then if accozding to the cōmon
maner thou haue recourſe to the humours, & bare qualities, and
ſo to ſéeke out and diſcerne the cauſes & oziginals of ſickneſſes,
by a certaine witty contemplation, rather then by that which is
moze true and infallible.

Thus we haue thought good to ſet down theſe things by way
of anticipation, concerning the exact and internall anatomy of humours, & concerning alſo the artificiall examining of them : both
that thereby it might appeare from whence the naturall impreſſions of things, & the infallible cauſes of diſeaſes are to be ſought,
as alſo that the true Philoſophers & Phyſitians may vnderſtand
thereby the way to cōpound prepare, and adminiſter artificially
medicines and remedies, which now we intend to ſhew, euen
accozding to the ozder and methood of the Dogmatickes. So as
wée thinke it not good, vtterly to reiect the olde, noz wholy
to followe the newe, but to reſtoze the old fozme of compoſiti-

on

on of Medicines increafed and amended with many of our inuentions, experiments, and compofitions, for the publique good, and for the health of the ficke , as alfo for the inftruction of fome ignorant Phyfitians.

An Elixir of our defcription.

A wonderfull remedy to cure inueterate and almoft defperate difeafes, and to conferue health, and to prolong life, as followeth.

Take of the roote of Zedoary, of Angelica, of Gentian, of Valerian , Tormentil , or Setfoyle, Goates beard, Galanga, the wood Aloes , and citrine or yeallow Sanders , of each three Ounces. Of Baume, of red Mint, Matoran, Bafil, Hyfope, Germander, Chamepithis, of each halfe a handfull: of Lawrell Berries & Juniper, of the feedes Peony, of Sefeli, or Comin, of Anis, of Mugworr, of Cardus-Benedictus, of each two ounces : the barke of Citrine, of Miffel of the oake, and of all the Mirabolans, of each one Ounce. Cloues, Cinamum. Mace, Ginger, Cubebs, Cardamony, Pepper, long and round, Spikenard, of each one ounce and a halfe. Aloes Hepat, Myrrhe, Olebanum, Maftic, of each fixe Drachmes . The flowers of Rofemary , of Sage, of Stechades, of Mary golds, of Saint *Ihons* woort, of centaury the leffer, of Betonie, of the Linden tree, of each fo many as yee can gripe with two fingers and the thumbe at twife : of the flowers of Chicory, commonly called Suckary, of red Rofes, and of Bugloffe, of each one gripe in like fort onely, of grust hony, and of white Suger, of each one pound. Of *Aqua-Vitæ* after the beft maner rectified ten pound. Cut that which is to be cut, and beate that which is to be beaten.

All thefe things being put into a large Matrat, and clofe ftopt that no breath come foorth, fet in horfe-dung meanely hote, by the fpace of eight or ten dayes, to putrifie.

Being putrified, let them be hard and well preffed or ftrained, and put the liquor diftrained into an Allembic, and diftill it by a Cornute, at aconuenient fire.

The firft water which commeth foorth from the diftrained liquor,

liquor wil be moſt cleare : kéepe it by it ſelfe for it is precious,

Thy Receiuer being of glaſſe muſt be of good receit, and muſt be paſſing wel cloſed with the Cornute by the necke, that the leaſt vapour come not forth. And when the Recepuer beginneth to bée darkened, and to be filled with white ſpirits, thou ſhalt increaſe thy fire by degrées a little and a little, according to arte, vntil the ſaid whited ſpirits appeare no more.

The water of 2.degree. Mercurie.

Then take away the Receiuer, that thou mayſt put by it ſelf that water which commeth forth the ſecond time, and kéepe it wel : it is called the mother of Balſam, being very profitable to roote out many ſickneſſes, and to conſerue health.

An Oyle. Sulphur, Fyer.

Then againe put to thy Recepuer, and increaſe thy fire by degrées, as thou didſt before, ſo long vntil at the firſt, there diſtill forth a yealow oyle : after that a red oyle, the matters in the Matrad remaining drie : and yet not throughly drie, leaſt the liquor which ſhall diſtil forth doe ſmel of burning.

Theſe things done, take that moſt cléere water which came forth firſt of all in good plentie : powr it vpon the feces remayning : and make them to digeſt together by the ſpace of 6. or 7. dayes, at the heate of *Baln-marie*, vntil the water be coloured and waxe yellow : that is to ſay, vntill it hath attracted the more fierie and oylie portion of the matter : and the feces which ſhall remaine, when they haue yéelded their whole tincture to the foreſaid water, reſerue and kéepe apart to ſuch vſe as herafter ſhal be declared.

The Feces, Salt. Earth,

(But if you think good, you may reſerue a portion of euery of the ſaid liquors to ſuch medicinable vſes as is before ſhewed, and vſe the reſt in the progreſſe of the foreſaid worke. and in the ſubſequent.)

After you haue drawne the foreſaid liquors, & that alſo which tooke laſt tincture from the feces, thou ſhalt mixe them together, that from thence thou mayeſt extract a farre more *Elixir* of life, than the former, and moſt precious : procéeding in manner following.

When thou haſte mixed the foreſaid thrée liquors together, thou ſhalt diſtil them by a Cornute, or by a glaſſe Allembic, pretermitting

A moſt precious Elixir,

termitting al digeſtion, vſing no other than the ſayd mixture: vſe
and follow the ſame way & order, which thou diddeſt before, ſeperating the Elements, and beginnings of liquors.

For thou ſhalt draw out of the firſt moſt cleare water, which
thou ſhalt reſerue by it ſelfe, namely, at ſuch time as thou ſhalt
perceiue the receiuer to be darkened with a cloudie fume : then
chaunging the Receiuer, and putting to fire as thou didſt before, thou ſhalt continue it ſo long, vntil thou ſée the liquor to iſſue
forth of yealow colour, the which alſo thou ſhalt kéepe apart as
thou diddeſt the former.

In the meane time while the foreſaide diſtillations, or ſeperations of Elements, that is to ſay, of the two beginnings,
Mercurie and Sulphur, are in hand, thou ſhalt calcine, at a
Reuerberatorie fire, the Feces which thou reſeruedſt before :
out of the which, being brought to aſhes, thou ſhalt extract ſalt,
according to Arte, with thy firſt moſt cleare water; the water
ſeaſoned with his Salt, ſhal be mingled with the other two liquors which were reſerued, that ſo at the leaſt out of a Try-
angle, thou mayeſt make a Circle O, as Philoſophers ſpeake:
that is to ſay, that out of thoſe thrée ſeueral waters, by circulation (in a Pellican) made according to Arte, there may come
forth one eſſence : and ſo by that meanes that great *Elixir* of
life, and admirable ſecret ſhal be made.

And not onely made, but alſo by ſo ſhort a way, ſo eaſie, and
ſo well knowen to true Philoſophers, that they know thereby, how, and in what order to make *Elixirs* out of all
things.

The vertues of this *Elixir* are vnſpeakable, both to the curing & alſo to the preuenting of giddineſſes in the head, the Falling ſickeneſſe, Apoplexies, Palſies, madnes, Melancholy, the
Aſthma, and diſeaſes of the Lungs, faintings and ſoundings,
traunces, weakeneſſe of the ſtomach, and of other parts, conſumptions proceeding of an euil diſpoſition of the bodies, paſſions proceeding from the gaule, and ſuch like heauie and lamen-
table griefes.

Certaine droppes onely of this, being giuen in ſome conuenient

nient breath, and fitting for the ſickneſſe. As for example, againſt the Epilepſie, with water of Peonie; of Lillies, Connally, or of flowers of the Linden trée. Againſt the palſie, with the water Mary golbes : againſt the peſtilence with the water of Coates beard, or of water of *Cardus Benedictus* : againſt the Aſthma or Tiſſick, with the water of Scabioſe, or of Fole-foote, or ſuch like.

Moreouer this *Elixir*, is of force to reſtore and conſerue our radial Balſam, if fewer or fine droppes thereof, be giuen in broath, wine, or other conuenient liquor.

But peraduenture thou wilt ſay, that the preparation of this *Elixir*, requireth too much labour, & is too tedious. But it is much better and more neceſſarie to ſpend the time in things ſo admirable and of ſo great importance, than about Medicines that are altogether vnprofitable. And yet to ſerue euery mans turne, I wil ſet downe the preparation of an other *Eilxir*, more eaſie, and peraduenture more pleaſing, to conſerue health, and to prolong life.

Another Elixir of life moſt eaſie to be made.

TAke the Rootes of *Gentian* ſlit in pieces, and dryed with a gentle heate, alſo the roote of the leſſer Centaurie, of each thrée ounces. Galanga, Cinimon, Mace, Cloues, of each one ounce. Flowers of Sage, of S. *Iohns woort*, of each two grypes with two fingers and a thumbe. Of the beſt white wine 6. pound. Infuſe theſe in a glaſſe Matrate, wel ſtopped, by the ſpace of eight dayes, at a gentle fire of *Balne-Marie*. Then let them be wel ſtreined, & ſo diſtilled by a glaſſe Allembic in aſhes, til nothing remaine but dryneſſe.

Then powre the water diſtilled vppon the feces, that from them thou mayeſt drawe away the whole tincture, in a milke warme *Balne-Mary*: Bring the Feces (after the drawing away of the tincture) into aſhes, which thou ſhalt put into *Hyppocrates* bag, powring the ſaid coloured water oftentimes vpon the aſhes, that it may draw vnto it the proper ſalt.

Giue of this *Elixir* the fourth part of a ſpoonefull in ſome conuenient liquor. Uſe it a long time. It is a ſpecial remedie for all conſumptions, for the weakneſſe of the ſtomache , which

Hippocrates bagge, is like the bagge where through Hypocras runneth.

it

it purgeth from tough and ſlimy humours which cleane to the ſame : It ſtayeth the bꝛeeding of woꝛmes, and keepeth the body in health. Take of this twiſe in one weeke and continue with it.

A *Treacle water* for the head, helping all paines of the ſame, proper for the Apoplexie, Epilepſie, Palſey, and ſuch like.

Take of the rootes of Peony, of Miſſelto, of common A-coꝛns oꝛ Cane, of each thꝛee ounces. Of ripe Junipar-berryes, and of the ſeeds of Peony, of each, one ounce : Of Cloues and Maces, of each 6. dꝛachmes. Of Caſtoreum, halfe an ounce : Of the flowers of Stechados, Mary-gold, Roſe-mary, Sage, Lillyes conually, of the Linden tree, of each, two grypes with two fingers and the thumbe. Cut that which is to bee cut, and beate that which is to bee beaten : and infuſe them by the ſpace of 9. dayes, by the heat of a hote Balne, in white wine of the beſt, 2. pound: and with the waters of Peony, Sage, and of Mary-goldes, of each one pound.

Then ſtraining them hard. To this liquoꝛ adde of Treacle of Alexandꝛia, ounces 4. of *Anacardine confectionem Meſu*, one ounce and a halfe, of *Diamoſch*, and *Aromatici Gabriel*, of each halfe an ounce.

Steepe oꝛ infuſe theſe againe, by the ſpace of two oꝛ thꝛee dayes, at the fire gentle of *Blan. M.* Then ſtraine them againe, and diſtil them vpon aſhes to dꝛineſſe : and thereof a Treacle-water wil bee made.

A very ſmal ſpoonefull of this is ſufficient to be giuen at once againſt the diſeaſes befoꝛe expꝛeſſed.

Another Treacle-water cordiall, and comfortable for the heart, very good againſt al peſtiferous effects therof vſed, with great profite.

Take of the rootes of *Angelica*, of Cloues, of Goates beard, of Toꝛmentil oꝛ Set-foyle, of Bifolium, oꝛ two-blades of

Enula

Enula campane, of each two ounces. Of yealow Sanders, and of the barke of the fame, of each one ounce and a halfe. Of white Diptani, of Scabiole, of Rue, of Goates beard, otherwiſe called Madwort, of each one handfull. Of the Flowers of the leſſe Centaure, of S. *Iohns-woort*, of Bromme, of Violets, of Borage, of Bugloſſe, of Water-Lyllie, of Red Roſes, of each, a three finger gripe. Put theſe into 3. pound of Malmſie infuſed by the ſpace of 4. dayes, ſet vpon the fire of *Baln M.* and the Iuice of Lemons, the water Meliſſa, Acetouſe, and of Roſes mingled with the ſayd Wine, of each one pound. Then ſtrayne them.

In the liquor diſtrained, put of Treacle ounces three, of the confection of Viacinth, one ounce. Of the confection Alchermes, 6. drachmes. Of Diamargarit friged, Diatria Santali, of each 3. drachmes : of Diambre, and Diacoral, of each two drachmes, of Saffron, and Myrrhe, of each halfe a drachme.

Infuſe them againe, by the ſpace of two or three dayes, at the ſame fire of *Baln. M.* Then diſtil them to drineſſe by fire of aſhes: and it will be a Treacle water. But to make it the more effectuall, the Salt muſt be extracted out of the feces which remaine, according to arte, and then mingeled with the foreſaid water.

A water againſt Poyſons, and againſt all peſtilentiall effects.

Take of the Rootes of *Angelica*, of the Carline-thiſtle, of Set-foyle, & of the Barke of the Olibian Tree, of each two ounces, of *Cardus Benedictus*, of Made-wort, called Goates beard, of all the Sanders, of each halfe an ounce: the Treacles of Mythridate, and the confection of Viacinth, of each 2. ounces: the ſpeces of Diamarg. Frigid, Camphor, of each 2. Drachmes. Let theſe be groſſely beaten or bruſed, & put into a glaſſe Allembic, powring thereon 3. pound of rectified *Aqua vitæ*. Then let them be digeſted in a veſſel wel cloſed, & ſo diſtilled by aſhes, or a vaporous *Baln.* This water is wonderfull effectuall againſt poyſonful and peſtilential effects. The quantitie which muſt be giuen, is halfe a ſpoonfull.

An

An excellent water to be giuen againſt Feuers, burning
and peſtilentiall.

Ake of the rootes of *Angelica, Bugloſſe, of Scorzonera A-*
cety, one ounce: of the Treacle Alexandzine, 2.ounces: of
the Iuice of Lemons clenſed, of the waters Fumetarie,
Gotes beard, and *Cardus Benedictus*, and of the leſſer centaure,
of each, ounces 4. *Diamarga, Frigid,* halfe an ounce. Let theſe
lye infuſed by the ſpace of thzœ oz 4. dayes: then let them be diſtrained and diſtilled Of the which let the ſicke dzinke 4.ounces:
and then being well couered in his bed, he ſhal ſweate moze than
ozdinary.

Principall Remedies to eaſe the torments and extreame
paines of the *Goute.*

Ake of the leaues of Miſſel, which groweth on the Apple-
trœ, cut oz ſhzed very ſmal, halfe a pound: the flowers of
white Mulline, of Chamomil, of Lyllies, of Wallwozt, oz
Danewozt, all the kindes of Poppey, with their caſes which
containe the ſœd, new gatheres, and befoze they be full ripe, of
each one gripe of the 2. fingers and the thumbe, of grœne Frogs,
oz in ſtœd of them, the Jelly oz ſperme of Frogges, which is to be
found in ſtanding waters in the Moneth of March, one pound:
the ſœd of white Poppey bzuſed, 4. ounces: of Crabbes oz Cra-
fiſhes ſhelles, and all beaten oz cruſhed together, 20. in number: of red Snailes, and Earth-wozmes, both wel waſhed in
good white wine, of each 4. ounces: of Badgers greaſe ſire
ounces; of Sperma Ceti, 4. ounces: of the oyle of violets oz water Lilly, newly made, 6 pound: oz if you wil, in ſtœde of theſe
oyles, take ſo much of oyle Oliue.

Put theſe into a glaſſe veſſel, foz that purpoſe conuenient,
and cloſe ſtopt ſet it in hozſe dung by the ſpace of 7. oz, 8. dayes.
But if need require moze haſte, let them boyle in a Copper veſſel
ouer the ſire, by the ſpace of two houres, and then ſtraine them
ſtrongly. The which alſo you ſhalt doe, if they ſtand in Hozſe
dung to be digeſted.

Thos

Thou then ſhalt ſeperate the oyle from the watery part thereof accoꝛding to arte: to the which oyle, thou ſhalt adde of Saffron 2. ounces, of Camphyꝛe, hale an ounce.

Put all theſe into a glaſſe veſſel, and ſet them againe in Hoꝛſe
dung, oꝛ in Balneo, oꝛ in the Sunne, by the ſpace of 5. dayes,
and thou ſhalt haue a moſt excellent Balſam to aſſwage and qua-
liſie all paines of the Goute, and in the ioynts.

I wiſh that all Apothecaries would pꝛepare this, to be rea-
ry at al times foꝛ pꝛeſent vſe: foꝛ that they cannot appoint themſelues of any thing better than this, which my ſelfe haue found
true by experience.

A plaiſter to helpe and eaſie all paines of the Goute.

Take the marrow oꝛ pulpe of Caſſia foure ounces, of new
Treacle, the newer the better, halfe an ounce. The meale
of Barley and Oates, of each thꝛée ounces. The crumbes
of white bꝛeade foure ounces: of Cowe-milke, two oꝛ thꝛée
pound.

Let al theſe be ſodden in the foꝛme of a Cataplaſme, which
thou ſhalt apply warme to the grieued parts. If thou ſhalt adde
one ounce of vitriol calcined, and beaten into fine pouder, thou
ſhalt make it much better.

Another Cataplaſme.

Take the diſtilled water of whyte Mulleyn, and of Ferne, of
each halfe a pound: of calcined vitriol as befoꝛe, one ounce
and a halfe: of Oate-meale 4. ounces: Of Saffron two
dꝛachmes, make a Cataplaſme.

A water againſt the paine of the Coute.

This water following pꝛepared in due time, will much auaile
againſt the greateſt paines of the Gout, where there appeareth redneſſe, and much heate.

Take of the diſtilled water of the ſperme of Frogges, of
Nightaper & of Ferne, of each one pound and a halfe. In theſe
inſuſe Tuttie, and Lytharge, of each two ounces: Vitriol calcined
and Allum, of each one ounce. Let the grieued parts, be moyſtened with linnen cloutes wet in the ſame, applyed warme, renuing
the ſame diuers times.

An

Another excellent water againft the Goute.

Take of the Sope of Genua, that which is white and good, one ounce. Of liquid Salt, made to runne at a ftrong fire, one ounce and a halfe: of Vitriol, one ounce: of Acatia, halfe an ounce. Let them all boyle together in a pinte of Rofe vinegar, or of common vinegar. With this liquor wafh both the greiued partes.

An excellent playfter, which being layed vpon the knots and puffes of the Gout, diffolueth them.

Take of the oyle of Apple Miftel, of our defcription, one or two pound : warme it in a veffel at the fire : being made warme, put into it of fhaued or fcrapings of Sope 4. ounces, let them be well ftirred together with a fpattle, vntil the oyle and Sope bee wel incorporated together. After this, put thereto *Venis Ceruſe*, and *Lytharge*, of each 2. ounces, euer mingling and ftirring them with a fpattell: of Vitriol calci-ned til it be red, and pouldred, one ounce. Of Cinabar halfe an ounce. When any of the aforefaid things are put in, ftirre it wel til it come to a conuenient thickneffe for a playfter : which thou fhalt apply to the knots : it helpeth not onely thefe, but alfo al cal-lous, and hollow vlcers and pockes.

An excellent water to the fame effect.

Take Vnflickt-Lime, let it lye in Spring water fiue or fixe dayes, that thou mayeft draw out the Salt. Let the water be foure or fiue fingers aboue the Lyme. Of this water take 3. pound : in the which thou fhalt quench a red hote plate of Stéele, twelue times, and oftener.

After this, thou fhalt put therein of burnt copper brought into ponder 3. ounces: of Cinabar, halfe and ounce. Let them ftand by the fpace of foure or fiue dayes, in which time the water will be of a gréene colour, by meanes of the inward vitriol of the burnt copper. This water is an excellent remedy to qualifie and alay fuddenly all manner aches and paines.

A remedie:

A remedy to diſſolue the Stone.

After ſome conuenient gentle purgation, let the patient grieued with the Stone, take one little ſpoonefull of this poulder following, which not onely openeth the conduits prouoking vrine, but alſo diminiſheth and hindereth the growing of the Stone.

Take of the kernels which are in Medlars, of Gromel, called Milium Solis, the ſeedes of the great Burre, Sarifrage, Hollyhock, Anis ſeedes, Fennel-ſeedes, of each three drammes: of Chriſtall ſtones and of Tartar, ſix drammes: of the ſtones which are called commonly Crabbes eyes, halfe an Ounce, of the Salt of ground Furze, one drachme: of Cinamon one Ounce and a halfe: of Violated Suger, two Ounces and a halfe: mingle theſe and make a poulder. This poulder being taken, let the partie drinke vpon it, a little wine Juniperated, or of this water following.

Take of the rootes of Eryngium, of ground Furze, and of the fiue rootes apertiue, of each one Ounce : of the barke of *Lemons*, one Ounce and a halfe : of the foure greater cold ſeedes, of the ſeedes of Mallowes, and Hollihock, of each three Ounces, of the ſeedes of Sarifrage, of Gromel, of the greater Radiſh, of the Burdock, and of ripe Junipar Berries, of each, Drachmes ſix : of Alkakeng Berries, twenty in number, of Juiubes ſix couple, of Dictam, of the flowers of Broome, of Saint *Iohns* wort, of Betonie, of the greateſt Mallow, of each two gripes with the thomb and two fingers: of liquirice, two ounces and a halfe: of the wood of *Caſſia*, one Ounce: beate and poulder that which is to be pouldered: and let them be ſteeped or infuſed in water of ſiluer weed, called wilde Tanſey, and of Parietory of the wall, of each one pound and a halfe : of the beſt white wine two pound, and that by the ſpace of foure daies, in Bal. *M.* hote : and then let it be ſtrongly ſtrained.

Into the liquor, put of the Species of Diatragaganthum Frigidum, and of the Trochiſces of Alkakenge, without Opium,

of

of each one Ounce . Let them be digefted againe at the fire or Baln.Mar,by the fpace of one oz two dayes:and let them be dif-tilled by a glaffe Allembic,accozding to Art. This water alfo ta-ken by it felfe alone , cutteth and thinneth groffe matters,and clenfeth the raynes and fucking vaines , and the bladder,from the ftopping of fand and grauel , and freeth them from groffe humours.

Of this water by it felfe alone,the dofe to be giuen at one time is two Ounces, with fome conuenient fyzrup.

An other excellent water againft the Stone.

TAke the Juice of Radifh,of *Lemons*,of each one pound and a halfe,of the waters of Betonie, of wild Tanfey, of Sari-frage,of Veruaine,of each one pound:of Hydzomel,and of Malmefey,two pound. In thefe liquozs mixed together,infufe by the fpace of foure oz fiue dayes at a gentle fire of Baln. Mar, Junipar Berries ripe and newe gathered, being bzuifed,thzee Ounces,of Gromel, of the feede of the Burdock, of the greater Radifh,of Sarifrage,of Nettels,of Onions of Anis,of Fenel,of each one Ounce and a halfe, the foure cold feedes, the feedes of great mallowes, of each fix dzachmes: the fpecies of Lithon tri, the Electuarie *Duis & Iuftini Nicolai*,of each halfe one Ounce : the Calxe of Egge-fhels, Cinamon, of each thzee Dzachmes,of Camphoze two Dzachmes,Let all againe be well diftrained and then diftilled by afhes.

Two ounces of this water taken , doth wonderfully clenfe the Counduits , pzouoke bzine , and wil bzeake and expell the Stone. To this if you adde his pzoper Salt,oz one fcruple of the extract of Betonie,it will be a moze effectuall remedy.

The

The conclusion of this Treatise.

ALchymie oʒ Spagyꝛick, which fome account among the foure pillers of medicine, and which openeth and demon-ſtrateth the compoſitions and diſſolutions of all bodies, together with their pꝛeparations, alterations, and exalta-tions, the fame I fay is ſhe which is the inuenter and Schoole-miſtreſſe of diſtillation.

Foꝛ *Alchymie* vſeth feuen woꝛkes, which are as it were cer-taine degrees, by which as it were by certaine neceſſary inſtru-ments, ſhe oꝛdereth and finiſheth the tranſmutations of things. By tranſmutation I meane, when any thing fo foꝛgoeth his out-ward foꝛme, and is fo changed, that it is vtterly vnlike to his foꝛ-mer fubſtance and wonted foꝛme, but hath put on another foꝛme, and hath aſſumed an other eſſence, another colour, another ver-tue, and another nature and pꝛoperty. As foꝛ example, when lin-nen rags are turned into paper: metall into glaſſe: ſkins oꝛ leather into glue: an hearbe into aſhes: aſhes into Salt: Salt into water, and Mercury fo moueable, into a fixed body, as into Sinabar, and poulder.

The feauen degrees of working are thefe mentioned be-fore in the Practife.

1	Calcination,	Which is the bꝛinging of any thing to aſhes.
2	Digeſtion,	Is a diſſoluing of that which is thick in-to thinne, to be purified.
3	Fermentation,	Is a mixing of kindly matter foꝛ multi-plication, oꝛ the kindly feafoning, oꝛ leauining of a thing.
4	Diſtlliation,	Is an extraction of a liquoꝛ from a bo-dy, by heate.
5	Circulation,	Is to rectifie any thing to a higher per-fectioa.
6	Sublimation,	Is the lifting vp of moyſt matter, to make it moꝛe pure and dꝛy.
7	Fixation,	Is to make that which is flying, to a-bide with his body.

Befids

Beſide theſe, there are diuers other workings, as

- Diſſolutiõ, is to diſſolue ẙ which is groſſe.
- Putrifaction, is the meane to generation.
- Exaltation, is euaporation of the impure humour.
- Rectification, is a reiterated Diſtillation to perfection.
- Coagulatiõ is the congealing of moiſture.
- Cohobatiõ, is a repetition of Diſtillation, by which the liquor diſtilled is powred vpon the feces, and diſtilled againe.

Diſtillations are diuers , accoꝛding to the diuerſities of reaſons, maners, and of ſubiects : whereupon ariſe ſundꝛy differences of diſtillation.   The firſt difference is taken from things, out of which a moiſture oꝛ liquoꝛ may be dꝛawne. Foꝛ after one maner Hony: after another, Sulphur: after another Wine: after another Waxe: after another Turpentines and Gummes, as Maſtic, Euphoꝛbum, Styꝛax, and ſuch like: after another, Salts; after another Yearbs : after another, Rootes : after another many ſeedes are to be diſtilled.

The ſecond difference is taken from the diuerſitie of the liquoꝛ diſtilled. Foꝛ waters, are otherwiſe extracted then are oyles. As foꝛ example, out of Yearbes, Rootes , Flowers and ſeedes, which are not dꝛy, but growing, waters are extracted by ſimple diſtillation, without the admixture of any other liquoꝛ. But out of Rootes, Yearbes, Flowers, and ſeedes which are dꝛy and odoꝛiferus, the floating oyles are not extracted, without the meanes of ſome water oꝛ other liquoꝛ as a helpe.

The third difference dependeth vpon the matter and faſhion of the veſſels. Vpon the matter: foꝛ one veſſel is of earth, another of bꝛaſſe, another of lead, another of glaſſe.

Vpon the faſhion alſo : foꝛ there is one maner of diſtillation by an Allembic, another by a Coꝛnut, another by a Matrat, and another by a Pellican, and ſo of others.

The fourth difference is by the ſite and placing of the veſſell.

Foꝛ

For if it be by a right Cucurbit, which hath a head with a pipe or beake, or whether it be inclining or crooked, we call ſuch diſtillations, by aſcent : or when the neck of one Matrate or cucurbit, is put into the neck of another, that is to ſay, whē the veſſels by concourſe are ſo ioyned together, that one taketh in the mouth of the other, and the ſame by a diuers poſition : and by theſe moſt commonly are diſtilled thoſe things which doe hardly aſcend, and haue ſmall ſtore of iuice.

Many things alſo are diſtilled by diſcent, that veſſell which containeth the matter turned the wrong way, and put into the other, the which manner of working is called by Diſcent, and is contrary to that which is by Aſcent.

By Diſcent are diſtilled Ceates, and ſundry kinds of fat wood, as Giraiacum, Junipar, and thoſe of roſen ſort.

The fifth difference is, by the degrees of fire, which are foure: the firſt, ſecond, third, and fourth.

The firſt is ſoft and gentle, ſuch is the fire of Balne. Mor of vapour: the ſecond, is of aſhes : the third is of ſand, or of the duſt of yron that falleth from the Smithes hammer in his worke at the Stythee. The fourth is of bare fire.

By the firſt and ſecond degree of fire, we diſtill by Aſcent: by the third and fourth, we diſtil by concourſe and Diſcent : Thus oyles are diſtilled out of Salts, as out of common Salt, out of Vitriol, and out of ſuch like.

But before you begin to diſtil, be ſure that you diſſolue & putriſie.

But becauſe mention is made before of Digeſtion and Fermentation, I will ſhew you plainly, how by theſe two meanes you may extract out of Roſes a moſt Fragrant water of life, and ſo excellent, that one droppe thereof, ſhall giue a ſweete ſent and odour to a great quantity of common water, and wil alſo make the the ſame moſt profitable and ſweete.

Therefore take Roſes gathered in due time, when there is neither raine nor deawe vppon them, but tarry till the Sunne with his beames hath diſpearſed and taken away that humiditie. Gather then of them a good quantity: and then bruiſe or beate them in a ſtone morter, or elſe

thou

Thou shalt put them into a small bostet of oake , and shalt with diligence presse them in with thy hands, in such sort that the vessell may bee stuffed ful almost to the toppe . Then stoppe and close it vp, that Digestion may more easily bee made, and set in a wine seller by the space of one moneth, or longer if nœde require , vntill thou shalt perceiue that the foresaide matter haue the odour of tart wine : whereby thou shalt knowe that the Fermentation is perfected : and so long it must at any hand bee delayed vntill the foresaide signe doe appeare.

These things thus finished , take to thæ the fourth or fifth part of the Roses Fermented , according to the greatnesse of thy vessel, which necessarily must be such as the *Chymicall* Distillars doe vse wherewith they extract their oyles , and *Aqua-Vita*, the which indœde are large, and of Brasse, rather then of Lead, furnished with their refrigeatories (as they terme them) which being full of water, the spirits made thick through cold are more easily and commodiously drawen forth: Taking I say, that portion of Fermented Roses, distill them according to the wonted maner. That done, seperate the feces remayning, which subsist in the bottome of the Allembic, and put so much of the Fermented Roses aforesaid into the same vessell , and power vpon them the water extracted before , distilling altogether againe, vntill there appeare diuers ; thy vessell as well closed as may be as is said afore.

Gather againe the dryed feces (the which if thou wilt, thou maiest reserue with the former feces) and put the same quantity of the foresaide Roses into the Allembic which thou riddest before, vpon which againe thou shalt power all the distilled water: And this thou shalt doe so often vntill thou hast distilled all the said former t.o Roses.

These things orderly done, thou shalt take all the distilled water, and shalt distill onely the twelth part thereof, with a gentle fire in a vessell with a long neck or Matrate, or in such a one as *Aqua-Vita* is distilled, which is the quantity of all the spirituall almost. As for example, if thou haue twelue pound of water, thou shalt onely extract one pound, which wil be very odoriferus most

swæte

sweete, and spiritual, as ready to take flame, as is that which is extracted out of wine.

This water if thou wilt yet make of greater vertue, thou maiest rectified againe But the rest of the water which shal remaine in the bottome of the Allembic, will be more fragrant, and better then that which is distilled after the common maner: whereinto also thou maist convey his Salt and insert it, by bringing the foresaid feces to calcination, & meshing the same oftentimes through *Hypocrates* sleeve or bagge with water, whereby it shal more easily draw unto it, and retaine that Salt. After the same maner also thou maiest draw waters of life out of violets and other flowers, and especially out of them which are hote and odoziferus, as Rosemary Sage, Betonie: and such other like, which are better and more effectuall against sicknesses, then if they be made accoyding to the common order. The least quantity hereof will worke wonderful effects.

If our Apothecaries would acquaint themselues with these Concostions, Fermentations, and Digestions, and understand them aright, in their workings immitating nature after a certaine maner, they should be able to effect diuers commendable and profitable preparations. Yea it is not fitting the Apothecary alone to know these things, but for the Physitian also the commander and director of the Apothecarie, if he respect his humour and the health of his patient.

But these things at this day are little regarded, insomuch that many Physitians either neglect them, or else disdainfully contemne them, for that they know not what profit such preparations doe bring with them. And verily I doe not know, what should be the cause of such obstinate disdaine & wilful contempt, but meere ignorance: seeing it is well known that nothing is contemned, but of the ignorant.

And what wil not these mad Ignorants contemne, which doe also despise the preparations of Medicines? which administer nothing to their sicke patients, but those things which are crude, and full of impurities. They rather chuse obstinatly to goe forware in their error, both to their owne reproach, and dammage of the sicks, then rightly to followe holesome admoni-

tions

tions, leaſt they might be thought not to haue bene wiſe enough
befoze, and to haue learned moze knowledge of others.

Let them conſider the neceſſitie of our life, that they may
learne that the ſame hath conſtrained vs, to ſeeke the pzeparations of our meates, which are neceſſarie foz the ſuſtaining of our
bodies: in the pzeparing whereof, notwithſtanding, there is not
ſo great neceſſitie as there ought to be in the pzeparing of medicines foz our health.

Let them beholde the cozne which commeth out of the earth,
which is not by and by giuen crude as it is, foz food: but the chaffe
and the bzanne being ſeperated, it is bzought to flower: which as
yet is not ſo giuen to eate, but being firſt fermented oz leuened,
e wel kneaded oz wzought, it is baked, that it may be bzead fit foz
nouriſhment. Conſider well the fermentation, by which bzead is
made light, and fit foz nouriſhment: the lighter it is, the wholſom-
er it is, and the moze it is fermented the lighter it wil be. The
leſſe it is fermented, the heauier it is, and the moze vnholſome.
If this pzeparation goe not befoze, but that we onely make a
mixture of water and flower together, and ſo pzeſently thzuſt
it into the Ouen, in ſteede of bzead, thou ſhalt pzepare a
glutinous matter very hurtfull to nature. Doe you not ſee
how paſte a glutinous matter, and ſtarch, alſo are made onely with flower and water? What then thinkeſt thou will come
to paſſe in thy ſtomach and bowels, eſpecially in thoſe which are
moze weake, if ſuch be offered and taken? Surely ſuch as will
pzocreate matter to bzeede the ſtone, and wil be the ſeminary of
many diſeaſes.

So neceſſarie and pzofitable is this Fermentation, that
it is very behouefull foz an Apothecarie to knowe it: foz that
it doth attenuate euery ſubſtance, it looſeneth it from his body, and terreſtrial impurity, that it may afterwards be made
fit to bzing fozth the true radical Balſam, and the quickening ſpirit.

By the benefite of this onely Fermentation, are extracted
waters of life out of all vegetables whatſoeuer. After the ſame
manner, by this Fermentation and Leauen of nature, all the

humours

humours of our body are made thinne and ſubtiled. You know how in holy writ it is ſaid, that a little ſowre Leauen doth ferment the whole maſſe.

By the way of *Fermentation*, which conſiſteth in a certaine Acetoſus liquor of nature, our humours are made thinne and diſpoſed to excretion. And therefore there are certaine tart things which moue ſweates, albeit the ſame by the opinion of Phyſitians are cold.

Doe wee not ſee that women and ordinary Cookes haue attained this knowledge of Fermentation: and thereby prouide for ſicke perſons, Iellyes made of fleſh of foules, and ſuch like, to reſtore and ſtrengthen them in the time of their weakeneſſe?

And what are theſe but extracts? For the terreſtrial partes are ſeperated from the more laudable ſubſtance, which is more conuenient for the ſicke. And why doe not Apothecaries the like in compounding their medicines?

The nature of the ſicke man being now weakened, cannot abide crude and fulſome meate, but doth rather loathe them, and is more and more weakened by them. How much more will he be offended and hurt by medicines not rightly prepared nor ſeperated from their impure ſubſtance? Such impuritie muſt needs be a great hurt and hindrance, that the natural force of the Medicine, cannot encounter with his enemie the ſickneſſe, and ouercome him.

What ſhall we ſay then of thoſe Medicines, which haue not onely cruditie in them, but alſo ſome euil qualitie, and the ſame not ſeperated, or rightly prepared: or being corrected, may wee be bold to giue it? They are wont, (with griefe I ſpeake it) too much and too often, I ſay they are wont, I meane ſuch decocted, pouldred, and mixed Medicines, by no manner of other art prepared, to bring more griefe and paine to the ſicke (that I may ſay no worſe) than ſollace and helpe.

Therefore theſe kinde of preparations, concoctions, I ſay Digeſtions, and Fermentations, are not to bee deſpiſed or neglected. For if theſe things be done, they are done according to natures faſhion, which uſeth the ſame operations to the perfect

ripening

ripening of fruites, and all things elſe which it bꝛingeth foꝛth.
But let vs haſten to conclude this Treatize.

Ariſtotle in his fourth of *Meteors*, hath appointed thꝛæ *Pip-
ſias*, oꝛ kindes of concoction. The firſt he calleth *Pepamſis*, which
is the concoction of humour in moyſt ſæde, made by naturall
heate : And this is the meane of concocting, ripening, and of wa-
king of the ſædes of Plants, and of other things to grow, and
to bꝛing foꝛth plentie of fruite : and it is a woꝛke onely belonging to nature, which vſeth that quickening heate foꝛ an Inſtrument, which heate anſwereth the element of Starres in pꝛopoꝛ-
tion, as the ſayd *Ariſtotle* ſaith. Albeit Arte cannot immitate
this heate, yet it may tread in the ſteppes thereof.

The ſecond kinde of concoction, he calleth *Epſeſis*, oꝛ *Elix-
ation*, which is a concoction made by a moyſt heate of a thing
ir.difinitely exiſting in a humour.

The third and laſt is *Opteſis*, oꝛ *Aſſation*, which is the concoction of the ſame interminate, made by a dꝛy and ſtraunge
heate.

Theſe two laſt concoctions, are made eſpecially by Arte, concerning the moderation of which heates, wæ will hereafter
teach the diligent and induſtrious Apothecaries, I ſay induſtrious, and ſuch as follow the pꝛeſcrips of true Phiſitians and
Arte, not Pedlars and Sellers of Trifels, which rather deſire to make retale of Candels, Lanternes, and all Mercerie-
wares, and to fill their ſhoppes with traſh, than to follow the
woꝛkes of Art.

Therefoꝛe in ſtæde of liberal perſons, they are miſerable hier-
lings: Sowters they are, and not Artificers and louers of
Art, Marchants, and handy crafts men, ſetting their reſt vpon
pompe, pleaſure and gaine. I had rather ſæ an enemie in the
Cittie, then one of theſe baſe minded fellowes. Foꝛ Citizens
know how to beware of an open enemie : but how can a man beware of the falſhood and treacherie of theſe companions which
they bꝛing to paſſe either by ignoꝛance, oꝛ by mallice oꝛ elſe by
negligence : I ſay who ſhall take hæde of theſe, but he which ba-
niſheth them quits and cleane out of the Cittie.

I ſpeake

I speake of deceiuers, and such as falsly vsurpe the name and tittle of Apothecaries, professing that, and yet follow the Trade of Marchandise, and not of honest and good men, which are dilligent in their Arte, to whom this our labour pertaineth, and to whom these our studies and admonitions are dedicated, for the health of many, and for their praise and profite.

The auncient Physitians and men of the best sort, delt more warily and prouided better for themselues, had this arte in great honor, and therefore in their owne houses, they prepared medicines with their owne hands.

And wee also for our owne partes would bee loath that some of our secrets, should bee cast before these Hogges, and therefore wee commonly prouide, that they bee prepared in our Laboratorie at home by a skilfull workeman, whome wee direct and appoint for that purpose.

Not that wee might make thereby the greater gaine to our selues, but for the honour and praise of the Arte, and to our friends good, the which all these know, that know vs, and haue receyued the benefite from vs. But for this time these shall suffice.

For the Patterne of Furnaces and glasses apt and méete for Distillation, buy Maister *George Bakers* Booke our Countryman.

And if thou be desirous to procure glasses of all sortes for this Arte, thou mayst haue them at the Marchants hand, which sell such in their houses néere the *Poultery* in *London.*

The winde Furnace, must haue a hole beneath, one foote déepe inwarde, and one foote and a halfe vpward: and at that height a grate shall be layed, wherein the coales of fire must lie. Also at that height make another mouth, where at thou shalt put in the saide coales of fire: and aboute the same raise vp the walles round about ten Inches in height and there also lay two barres of Iron to set the Panne vppon, either for *Balneum Marie,* or for a dry fire.

To make thy nouriſhing Balne,

TAke chopt Hay and water, and put it into an earthen Pan, then ſet ouer it a Trencher with a hole in the middeſt, to anſwere the bottome of the glaſſe, which muſt come within two Inches of the water.

Concerning Hermes Seale, *and the making of diuers cloſiers of glaſſes.*

FIrſt thou ſhalt know, that of all faſtnings or cloſing vp of Glaſſes, that no vapours nor ſpirits goe forth, the *Seale of Hermes* is moſt noble : which is done in this manner following.

First, make a little Furnace, with the Inſtruments belonging. It muſt haue a grate in the bottome to make fire vppon. In the middſt of the Furnace ſhall be a hole, to put in the ende of a narrowe necked Glaſſe, ſo that the third part of the glaſſe be emptie. And if the hole of the Furnace be greater then the glaſſes necke, cloſe vp the hole with claye on euery ſide, round about, ſo as the mouth of the glaſſe haue ſome libertie. Let thy fire be as farre from thy glaſſe as thou canſt : and when thy coale fire is readie, put the Glaſſe nærer and nærer, by little and litle, till the mouth of thy glaſſe waxe red, as it were ready to melt. Then take the red hote tonges, and therewith wring or nippe the toppe cloſe together : whereby it ſhall be ſo cloſed, as if it had no vent before, or came ſo cloſed out of the Glaſſe-makers ſhoppe. But take hǽd when you haue ſo done, that you pull it not too ſuddenly out of the fire, leaſt the ſudden colde cracke the glaſſe, and marre all. Therefore abate it by little and little, and not at once.

And when thou wilt open the glaſſe, take a thride dipt in brimſtone or waxe, and wind it 6. or 7. times about the necke of the glaſſe where thou wouldeſt haue it to breake, and ſet it on fire with a ſmall waxe candle, and when it is burnt, powre a

drop

drop or two of cold water vpon it, and it will crack in the ſame place, that thou maiſt take it off.

Concerning the maner of making Lutes, where-
with to cloſe glaſſes.

THe ordinary Lutes wherewith to ſtop veſſels of glaſſe a-gainſt faint vapours, are theſe. Take quick lyme beaten to poulder as fine as may be, and ſearſed: temper it with the white of egs. Or elſe mix wheat flower with the white of egges, ſpred them vpon linnen cloath, and wrap it diuers times about the mouth or ioynts of the glaſſe.

Other Lutes, called *Lutum Sapientiæ*, made for the defence of ſtronger vapours, either to parget and lute the body of the glaſ-ſes, or to ſtop their mouthes, or looſe their ioynts: which are to be wrought cleare, ſmooth, and without knots or bladders: in maner following.

Take potters earth, with a forth part of ſhorne floxe added to the ſame: an eigth part of white aſhes, with a forth part of dry horſe-dung. All theſe wel beaten together with an yron rod.

This is the right compoſition of *Lutum Sapientiæ*. There be that doe adde to this compoſition, the poulder of brick, and of the ſcales beaten from yron, finely ſearſed.

And for the more conuenient drying of veſſels ſo luted and fenced, you ſhal bore certaine holes in a wooden forme, into the which put the neckes of thy glaſſes, that their bottomes and bodies may be dryed the better.

Another moſt excellent Lute for the like incloſer is made of glaſſe and Uermilion, of each like quantitie, poulered and ſearſed, then incorporated with verniſh, and a little oyle of Linſœde, and making the whole like a ſoft poulteſſe which is to be ſpread on a fine linnen cloath, wrap it about the mouth & ioynts of the glaſ-ſes, and ſo ſuffer them to dry in the Sunne. Which albeit, it is a long worke, yet it is moſt ſure. For this will ſerue againſt the ſtrongeſt vapours that are.

Alſo to compound a Lute, wherewith to make your Fornace

C c   that

The practiſe of

that it may not riue, oz chap, take chalke and potters clay, and a
quantity of ſand, wzought together with wollen ſloxe and hozſe-
dung, incozpozated as afoze.

　　Thus courteous Reader, I haue ſhewed thæ ſuch ſecrets in
this Art, as neither *Querſitanus, Iſacus, Hollandus,* noz any other
Phyloſopher, haue befoze publiſhed in pzint to my knowledge,
but haue come to my hands in paper and parchment copies.
If thou be induſtruous, & doeſt tread the right *Hermetical* path,
thou ſhalt by the meanes of theſe helps, ſo plainly ſet befoze thine
eyes without *Hieroglyphicks* and Riddels, to do thy ſelfe
and thy countrey good. Thus wiſhing to thæ, as
to my ſelfe, good ſucceſſe in all thy godly in-
deuours, I commend them and thæ,
to the Lozd.

FINIS.